The Placebo Effect in Healing

The Placebo Effect in Healing

Michael Jospe

Lexington Books
D. C. Heath and Company
Lexington, Massachusetts
Toronto

Library of Congress Cataloging in Publication Data

Jospe, Michael.
   The placebo effect in healing.

   Bibliography: p.
   Includes index.
   1. Placebo (Medicine). I. Title.
RM331.J67   615'.5   77-6582
ISBN 0-669-01611-x

Published simultaneously in Canada.

Printed in the United States of America.

International Standard Book Number: 0-669-01611-x

Library of Congress Catalog Card Number: 77-6582

*To my family: the Jospes, Traests and Matsons,
and in loving memory of Cynthia Ann,
Kaethe, and Felix.*

Contents

Acknowledgments   ix

Introduction   xi

Chapter 1   **A Historical Perspective**   1

Chapter 2   **The Physical Characteristics of the Placebo Itself**   9

Theoretical Explanations   9
Research on the Physical Characteristics of the Placebo Itself   11
Comments and Conclusions   14

Chapter 3   **The Laboratory Study of the Placebo Effect in Nonpatient Subjects and Placebos and Analgesia**   17

The Classical Conditioning Perspective   17
Effects of Placebos on Various Tasks in the Psychology Laboratory   20
Hallucinogenic Drugs and the Placebo Effect   22
Pain, Placebos, and Placebo Analgesia   25

Chapter 4   **The Psychology of Illness and the Ecological Validity of Placebo Experiments**   35

Chapter 5   **Studies of Placebo Effects in Clinical Situations**   41

Placebo Effects in Medicine and Surgery   41
The Placebo Effect in Psychiatry   43

Chapter 6   **The Search for the Personality of the Placebo Reactor**   59

Reasons for Studying the Personality of Placebo Reactors   59
The Research Literature   61
Summary of the Literature on the Personality of the Placebo Reactor and Some Comments and Conclusions   88

Chapter 7   Situational Analyses of the Placebo Effect   93

Demand Characteristics, Instructions,
    Instructional Sets, and Expectancy   93
Therapeutic Milieu: The Therapist-Patient
    Relationship and the Personality of the
    Therapist   102

Chapter 8   The Placebo Effect in Psychotherapy   109

Chapter 9   Perspectives on Some Methodological Problems
             in Placebo Research   129

Chapter 10   Some Further Theoretical Perspectives on the
             Placebo Effect   137

Chapter 11   Overview and Coda   147

             References   149

             Author Index   163

             Subject Index   167

             About the Author   171

Acknowledgments

John G. Darley and Norman Garmezy, both of the Department of Psychology, University of Minnesota, Minneapolis, have given enormous support and encouragement to my interest in the placebo effect. Professor Darley's confidence in me and in my interests in the unusual meant that on a few occasions he had to steer me away from trouble. It also meant, however, that I became very comfortable in being the broadly schooled psychologist I am today. Professor Garmezy, without doubt the most exciting teacher with whom I have ever been privileged to study, kept me on my toes and taught me many of the skills I needed to write this book. He watched and guided me on occasions when I got so carried away by the excitement of the topic that the suspension of my critical faculties became a temptation. Neither of these men is, of course, responsible for any errors, blasphemy or outrage that I have perpetrated in this publication. My clinical mentor and dear friend, Professor Robert Wirt, Director of the Division of Health Care Psychology at the University of Minnesota Health Sciences Center, encouraged me to take the time to complete this book for publication. I thank him for that and many other things.

I would also like to thank Professor Kenneth Walker, of Emory University School of Medicine, for checking the manuscript for medical accuracy and for his useful comments. At Lexington Books I enjoyed working with Ms. Betty Labine, who worked on editing the early manuscript with me, and Mr. Mike McCarroll, Vice President and General Manager, whose consistent encouragement and friendliness were appreciated. My friends Eric Gordon and Janice Keywell prodded and pushed me and taught me not to split infinitives. Eric braved my wrath when I disagreed with his textual criticisms even after I solicited them. Janice typed the manuscript and showed much patience in everything, particularly working through chapter 6, when we were both tempted to pull our hair out—and were probably excellent candidates for anxioloytic placebo therapy.

Finally, to my parents goes my deepest gratitude for all they have done to help me to discover an exciting life that I have been able to live.

Introduction

Healing is an ancient art, medicine a more recent science. Demons, evil spirits, infestation and pseudotherapy gave way to anatomy, chemistry, physiology, and the discovery of microbes in the course of medical progress. Science cast out the alchemists together with the witchdoctors and their demons. With the advent of Newtonian science, "If x, then y" and "If not x, then not y" displaced cabalistic incantations as the prescription for progress. What physicians could discover through trial and error or learn from their scientific colleagues and then apply in practice obviously became what constituted the science of healing. Specific, recognized causal factors and specific manipulations resulted in specific effects. Causality came to reign over mind and matter, but was that the whole picture?

With a certain arrogance born of the huge success of mechanistic science and a knowledge of what constitutes "scientific" therapy firmly in one's mind, it is easy to look back at ancient (and not so ancient) healing practices, folk medicine, and witchdoctoring and to dismiss all as just so much worthless quackery. One can, with hindsight, look back thousands, hundreds, or even tens of years, saying: "Well, we know better now!" This book will make apparent that since a whole residue of "nonspecifics" accounts for a greater number of therapeutic successes than one might comfortably care to admit, we do not know better to the extent we might think we do, or desire. In truth, modern medicine has made remarkable advances, and as is equally true, much of ancient medicine was useless. But we should not be seduced by parsimony into thinking that scientific medicine has, by being explicit about its independent variables, disposed of a number of other variables that often contribute to any observed therapeutic effect. The thought seldom occurs to us that our view of scientific therapy tends to be somewhat overidealized.

Ellenberger (1970, p. 47) has summarized what he perceives to be the differences between primitive and scientific therapy. In primitive healing, healers are much more than physicians; they are the foremost personalities of their social groups, whereas in scientific therapy, healers are specialists among many (nonmedical) others. Primitive healers exert their action primarily through their personalities, whereas the scientific therapist applies scientific techniques in an impersonal way. The primitive healer is primarily a psychosomatician treating many physical diseases by psychological techniques, but in scientific therapy there is a dichotomy between physical and psychic therapy. The primitive healer's training is long and exacting and often includes the experience of severe emotional disease that has had to be overcome in order to help other people, but in scientific therapy the training is purely rational and does not take into consideration the personal, medical, or emotional problems of the physician. The healer belongs to a school that has its own teachings and traditions diverging from those of other schools, whereas the scientific therapist acts on the basis of a unified medicine, which is a branch of science and not an esoteric teaching.

xi

These distinctions, as will be shown in this book, are more fancy than fact. (I should immediately point out that the preceding sentence reads: "*more* fancy than fact" and not "*mere* fancy," lest I be accused of gross iconoclasm, for perhaps now is the time merely to shake rather than shatter the idols.) The problem we encounter here is that what is prescribed as the most desirable way for therapy (or, for that matter, science) to proceed is mistakenly fantasized to be the way in which it actually does proceed. As will become clear in this book, *any* treatment effort, no matter how small, may produce at least some response that cannot be attributed to the specific independent variable(s) under consideration, and an argument for an intensified search for the nature of these variables will be presented. The effects of treatment are not restricted to the specific factors identified in the treatment setting. Other, nontreatment, nonspecific factors may be of enormous importance in treatment outcome. The search for their nature and parameters is no less important whether one views them, on the one hand, as nuisance variables that interfere with a comprehensive and more accurate evaluation of treatment efficacy or, on the other, as "bonuses" that can boost the effect of any treatment.

In order to be as precise and clear as possible about our terminology, some definitions will be introduced shortly. These will be followed by some brief glances at the history of therapeutics to allow a better perspective on the whole issue. An examination of studies conducted on the placebo effect will allow an appreciation of the fact that therapeutic outcomes in current practice are often as remarkable (in essence if not precisely so in form) as some of those presented in the historical outline. The purpose of this will be to show that the "scientific" aspects of therapy need to be cast in a less sacred light, one in which the importance of the psyche in the healing of soma and persons in the healing of both will be stressed more than they are now. Hopefully, another point will emerge: Nonspecific effects should be viewed as an indicator of the power of psychological factors in *any* therapeutic endeavor, rather than as an embarrassment indicating the ineffectiveness of physical methods of therapy. Scientific, modern medicine has reached the stage where it should be able to consider comfortably the role of nonmedical (i.e., physiologically nonspecific) aspects of treatment.

Definitions

The most outstanding word in the literature of nonspecific variables in therapy is *placebo*. This Latin word, meaning "I shall please," appears as the first word in the ninth verse of Psalm 114 in the Vulgate. As various writers have pointed out in the extensive etymological investigations of this word (e.g., Shapiro 1964a; Kissel and Barrucand 1964), "placebo" first meant a title for the form of certain Roman Catholic vespers for the dead. Through secularization, its meaning changed to "flattery," "courtesan," and other similar words expressing the gaiety of post-Renaissance European court life. Its first medical usage has been traced to *Quincy's Dictionary* of 1787, in which "placebo" meant simply "commonplace method or medicine." *Hooper's Medical Dictionary*, in 1811, described the word as meaning ". . . all medicine prescribed more to please the patient than for its therapeutic effectiveness." The word underwent several changes in definition after 1811. Currently, *placebo* is defined as "any therapeutic procedure (or that component of therapeutic procedure) which is deliberately given to have an effect on, or does have an effect on, a symptom, syndrome or disease, but which is without specific activity for a condition to be treated" (Shapiro 1963).

An important note here is that the definition does *not* include the phrase "inert substance," but rather states ". . . without specific activity for the condition to be treated." Thus we can see that placebos are not *of necessity* inert. A placebo may be an *active* one (noninert) or it may be *inactive* (inert). Active placebos contain active but incidental ingredients in order to mimic all the telltale side effects of the experimental substance or the therapeutic treatment. An *exact* placebo is one that mimics all the physical characteristics of the experimental substance or treatment. Any medical treatment, and any psychological treatment, may be a placebo insofar as it might have a therapeutic effect unrelated to the specific effect for which it is administered. Any mechanical, surgical, or other therapeutic technique (including all medications, whether topical, oral, or parenteral) may be a placebo.

Shapiro (1963) defined the *placebo effect* as "the changes produced by placebos or procedures acting as placebos." We need some clarification about what such "changes" are. In pharmacological research, *drug response* (the behavioral change of subjects on drug) is distinguished from *drug effect* (that portion of the behavioral change that can be attributed to the pharmacodynamic action of the drug). The former allows for the inclusion of nonpharmacological variables; the latter refers strictly to pharmacological ones. In the literature on placebos, we often find that the terms *placebo response* and *placebo effect* are used interchangeably; this practice should be avoided because it can cause confusion. The terms should be used analogously to the similar terms *drug response* and *drug effect*. Fisher (1970a) indicated with great clarity that when we use the term *placebo response*, we should be referring to "the behavioral change of subjects receiving placebo," whereas when we use the term *placebo effect* we mean "that portion of the behavioral change which can be attributed to the symbolic transaction of being given medication, as contrasted with the behavioral change due to mere passage of time, repeated testing, or other 'spontaneous' influences occurring while on placebo" (pp. 37-38). Fisher's definition of *placebo effect* includes the phrase "the symbolic transaction of being given medication," thereby narrowing somewhat the range of situations in which it could be applicable. Turning back to the definition of *placebo* given above, we can substitute "any therapeutic procedure... which is without specific activity for a condition to be treated," thereby leading to a definition of *placebo effect* that I think is preferable: That portion of the behavioral change that can be attributed to any therapeutic procedure that is without specific activity for the condition to be treated, as contrasted to the behavioral change due to mere passage of time, repeated testing, or other "spontaneous" influences occurring while on placebo.

Fisher (1970a, p. 38) mentioned the use of two more terms relating to the distinction between placebo effect and placebo response we have just made. *Placebogenic* variables are nonspecific variables that contribute directly to placebo effects. Variables such as positive set, for example, may enhance drug effects, provided that drug potency is not marked, since the more potent the drug, the less susceptible is the drug response to the influence of nonspecific factors. Placebogenic factors can interact with CNS drugs in a potentiating way. *Prognostigenic* variables are nonspecific variables that are associated with spontaneous change over time; drug-placebo comparisons will be minimized the more favorable the prognostic level. We shall discuss instances of the operation of both of these kinds of variables later on in this book.

A *positive placebo effect* occurs when a symptom or disease reacts favorably to a placebo; a *negative placebo effect* occurs when the opposite is true (i.e., side effects or worsening of the patient's condition due to the placebo). Kissel and Barrucand (1964) have rather ingeniously suggested the terms *nocebo* (Latin: "I shall hurt, harm") and *nocebo effect* for negative placebo and negative placebo effect, respectively. Since I prefer using this term, in this book *placebo effect* will therefore be used instead of *positive placebo effect, nocebo effect* instead of *negative placebo effect* (when side effects are noxious), and *nocebo* instead of *negative placebo*.

Placebos are often used as controls in the clinical evaluation of new drugs. In the context of drug evaluation, a *single-blind procedure* is one in which the patient does not know whether he or she is receiving an experimental or control substance (usually an inert placebo). A *double-blind procedure* is one in which neither the patient nor physician (or others treating or evaluating) knows to which group patients have been assigned. (The importance of double-blind procedures is quite apparent in the light of recent research on therapist expectancies, experimenter effect, demand characteristics, and so forth to which further reference will be made. In a later chapter we shall also discuss the relationship such factors as demand characteristics bear to the double-blind procedure as well as some limitations of, and alternatives to, the double-blind procedure.) A *triple-blind procedure* is one where a preliminary study with placebos is carried out, after which the placebo reactors are excluded for the definitive study that follows. This procedure is of dubious value: Even though its aim is to exclude or minimize placebo effects, they may still occur in as high a percentage of cases in the definitive study as occurred in the preliminary one.

The situation quite clearly amounts to the fact that there is no guarantee that a person who has not reacted to a placebo in one situation will not react to even an active pharmacological agent in another without any placebo effect.

As Lasagna, Laties, and Dohan (1958) have demonstrated, placebos can mimic many of the effects usually thought to be the exclusive property of active pharmacological agents. Some of these are: a *time-effect curve* (a peak or maximum effect), a *cumulative effect* (increasing therapeutic effect with repeated doses), *carryover effects* (persistence of effect after cessation of treatment), and an inverse relationship between efficacy of a placebo and the severity of a symptom (a more severe symptom responds less effectively).

The literature also shows many examples of tolerance sensitivity and idiosyncrasy to placebos, as well as increasing improvement with increasing dose of placebo (Shapiro 1963). Some patients (Vinar 1969) can become addicted to placebos and will show many of the formal traits of drug dependence including a tendency to increase the dose, an inability to stop taking the placebos without psychiatric help, an almost compulsive desire to take the placebos, and withdrawal or abstinence syndrome on sudden deprivation of the "medication."

These are the main terms we encounter in the literature on placebos. Other less frequently encountered terms will be defined in context, when necessary.

Why Examine the Placebo Effect?

The placebo effect, although not stumbled upon only yesterday, was until relatively recently almost completely neglected as an object of study per se. Its history has been extensively documented by Shapiro (1959; 1960; 1963; 1964a; 1964b; 1966; 1971a; 1971b). Early experimental investigations were carried out by many investigators, for example, the study by Lasagna, Mosteller, von Felsinger, and Beecher (1954), which stands as a classic in the field. Honigfeld's critical reviews of much of the then existing literature, which were published in 1964 (1964a; 1964b), were well integrated but not detailed. In 1961, the Third World Congress of Psychiatry was held in Montreal. A special symposium on specific and nonspecific factors in psychopharmacology was held. Its proceedings, edited by Rinkel (1963) were published as a separate volume from the proceedings of the Congress. At the 1966 Fourth World Congress of Psychiatry held in Madrid, increased recognition was given to the importance of nonspecific factors, and the proceedings of a symposium devoted exclusively to these were edited by Rickels and published in 1968 (Rickels 1968a). Shapiro's writing on the subject of the placebo has been extensive and of particular importance in documenting its history, with summarized and highly compacted statements of the results of the research. There is little doubt that Shapiro has been the outstanding scribe of the placebo effect; his role has not been an essentially critical one, however.

Among the most useful of the several hundred sources I have read and consulted were the proceedings of the Third and Fourth World Congresses of Psychiatry (Rinkel 1963; Rickels 1968a) and a book, apparently the only one ever written on the placebo effect (as opposed to edited collections of symposium proceedings), by Kissel and Barrucand (1964), members of the Faculty of Medicine at the University of Nancy, France. Their book, *Placebos et effet placebo en médecine,* is primarily a guide for the use of placebos, rather than a critical review of the literature, even though it contains 578 citations covering empirical and experimental as well as theoretical contributions to our knowledge of the field.

Unlike that of Kissel and Barrucand, this book will examine critically and attempt not only to integrate experimental investigations of the placebo effect in both medicine and psychotherapy (the latter presents a curious problem indeed), but also to account theoretically for its modus operandi. In my opinion a gap exists in the placebo literature at the present time. There are reviews of the experimental literature, and in some of these, mention is made of theoretical and experimental work to be integrated, so that we get a view of particular theoretical orientations, the way they are analyzed, and the techniques that are used in the research. The state of knowledge of the subject is such that we cannot deal only with theories that have themselves been advanced as explanations for the placebo effect. The scope must be broadened beyond this boundary by introducing additional theoretical and nontheoretical formulations from the general body of psychological literature. Some of these have a readily apparent relationship to the placebo effect, others do not. Some of them will be brought in to aid our conceptual grasp of the placebo effect itself. Others will serve another purpose, namely, that of better understanding the phenomena under consideration by doing what Deutsch and Krauss (1965) called "making multiple connections" between constructs (so that the constructs are not isolated from one another but are interconnected; hence the possibility of going from one to another by various routes).

Following a historical perspective on the placebo effect, we will start examining the experimental literature by first focusing on the physical characteristics of the placebo itself and examining whether the form, taste, and color of the placebo are significantly related to the effects obtained. The focus will then shift to the laboratory investigation of the placebo effect in nonpatient subjects, with particular emphasis on the classical conditioning perspective, effects of placebos on psychometric performance, self-report scales and perception, hallucinogenic placebos, and placebo analgesia. A chapter on placebo effects in clinical situations (including medicine and surgery, the use of placebos in psychiatry, and prognostic uses of placebos) will be followed by an extensive look at the personality of the placebo reactor and the question of whether such a person even exists. Such factors as demand characteristics, expectancy, and therapist characteristics will be examined in a chapter on situational analyses of the placebo effect, after which the placebo effect in psychotherapy will be subjected to some scrutiny. Perspectives on some methodological problems in placebo research will be followed by a chapter in which I shall attempt to tie together, by calling on a number of theoretical perspectives, some of the findings of the placebo literature and also suggest some lines that future research might follow. The final chapter will consist of a brief overview of the book and some concluding remarks about the problem.

The Placebo Effect in Healing

1 A Historical Perspective

People view health as being natural, sickness unnatural. It is health that the body takes for granted, just as its lungs take in air and its eyes light; quietly, health remains and survives as an inconspicuous part of one's feelings about the general well-being of life. But sickness often makes an alien intrusion, rushing, as if by chance, past the shocked mind and jolting into awareness a multitude of problems.

—Stefan Zweig

These words written in 1931 might, given our current understanding of disease, sound maudlin and exaggerated, but in historical perspective their truth is startling. The era of any active attempts at healing probably began when one Neanderthal or Cro-Magnon person found that by doing certain things, another's suffering was relieved. Some sort of physician-patient relationship undoubtedly existed (as evidenced by archeological findings) well before the beginning of recorded history. "Because health is the natural condition of man," Zweig wrote, "it does not explain itself and needs no explanation. But each sufferer will always try to find a meaning for his suffering." The wish to alleviate illness is probably as old as human history. Some writers have extended this notion even further back: Harrison (1963) has pointed out that the healing art is far older than the human species; for example, a cat burying its feces or a dog licking its wounds are probably practicing instinctive but useful curative and preventive medicine.

Zweig (1966) wrote that people could not understand the reason for illness and suffering. Pain was senseless and incomprehensible. Illness must have come from somewhere: Could it not have been sent by someone, or that the afflicted had harmed or angered someone—hence the illness came as a punishment? The gods who sent lightning and frost could just as easily send down illness and pain. From humanity's earliest beginnings, the appearance of disease had an inseparable link with religious feelings and thoughts. If the idea that a dog licking its wounds *is* practicing some sort of instinctive medicine is accepted, then, as Harrison (1963) said, the first blundering curative attempts made by people were by their very nature quite a step backward from the instinctive medicine of animals. However, in one sense a significant advance had been made, for human treatment was based on a hypothesis (albeit incorrect) of causation—that is, disease was due to infestation by devils or to curses by enemies. The gods, good or evil, Zweig (1966) wrote, sent illness, and only the gods could remove it: This

1

belief was a very firm one during the dawn of healing. Unaware of their own ability to discover cures, helpless, indigent, weak, and lonely people stood at the entrances to their caves and, ignorant of any other step to take, cried to their magic gods for help; they beseeched the benevolent gods not to forsake them and the bad ones to leave them. The only cures they knew were their cries for help, their magic incantations, and their sacrifices of appeasement. (Interestingly, at this stage of our discussion, we might jump ahead for a moment to note that in the chapter dealing with the personality characteristics of the placebo reactor, we shall see how some studies have found such people to be religious and regular church attenders.) The gods, however, did not listen to mere mortals who knew neither where the gods dwelt nor how to prove to them the good intentions of their atonement. In addition, mortals were uncertain that they were communicating with the gods in the best way. Most people could not discover, unaided, the answers to their questions. Others, wiser, knew the answers. In their need, people sought these wise persons to mediate between themselves and the gods. The wise ones were experienced and knew the necessary magic and utterances to placate the powers of darkness. In prehistoric times, and to a large extent even in today's world, this mediator was a priest, a witchdoctor, or a shaman.

At first, people tried to cure disease with magic incantations. The struggle for health was not a fight against a particular illness, but rather a struggle for god. All medicine had theological roots in the form of cults, rituals, and magic. Since medicine and theology were of a kind, the healing enterprise consisted of mysterious medical arts and not of science. Interestingly, for example, Asclepius was both hero and god of healing and, in the *Iliad,* a mortal. He was the "blameless physician" among whose children were Hygieia and Panaceia. Across all cultures, cures were ascribed to miraculous intervention and had to be performed in sacred places conducive to the spirit of the miracles and prayers. There was as yet no dichotomy between knowledge and belief: The relief of suffering could not occur without the intervention of spiritual powers or without rites, pledges, or prayers. The priests practiced their medical art, not their scientific knowledge. They possessed the secrets of the movements of the stars, the meaning of dreams, and the mastery of demons. Ordinary people could not learn these secrets, which were passed from one generation to the next only to the initiated.

This primitive unity was destined to dissolve. In order for healers to become independent and give practical assistance to the sufferer so that symptoms would be relieved, illness had to be rid of its divine origin. This change did not mean that healers were perceived by their patients to possess less mystique (a mystique that healers still possess to a large extent even today), but rather that the functions of doctor and priest, which had at first been combined in the same person, were gradually assigned to different ones and the two inevitably became rivals. Medicine gradually shed some of its supernatural trappings, and doctors began to combine magic with physical concepts in seeking natural causes for illness; material substance, usually assisted by magic, was what medicine was all about, and this was the way things stayed for millennia. From primitive times through the civilizations of Babylon, Greece, Rome, the Middle Ages, and even afterwards, the *normative* history of medicine, as evidenced by its therapeutic practices, was until relatively recently (eighty or ninety years ago) largely the history of the placebo effect (Shapiro 1960). Indeed, as Gallimore and Turner (1977) have said, "much of medical history . . . can be viewed as an archival testimonial to placebo therapy" (p. 47).

The variety of substances to which patients subjected themselves (or were subjected) for eons is legion. Many of these were nocebos. Treatments were primitive, unscientific, shocking, often dangerous, and, worst of all, for the most part ineffective. Only because of people's desperation and the misery of illness did physicians continue to be useful, respected, and usually honored members of society. What these treatments consisted of was almost a matter of "you name it, they did it!" Treatments simply knew no bounds of bizarreness (or was it ingenuity?). A crystallized tear from the eye of a deer bitten by a snake might have been rather more difficult to obtain than a few drams of eunuch fat, but both were used when available and the physician so desired. Although frogs were presumably abundant and more readily available than either source of the ingredients just mentioned, a frog's spermatic cord and fluid might still have been a little hard to excise. But blood (of every conceivable species), fur (likewise), bricks, stones, sand, human perspiration, hair, and bodily organs and fluids might possibly have been obtained with little more difficulty than we experience when we have our prescriptions filled at our local corner drugstore. In all likelihood, a modern physician would shun crocodile dung, cobra venom, bleeding, cupping, and leeching, but would the effects of these horrendous treatments differ considerably from those of such currently used ones as distilled water, sugar capsules, and the host of vitamin pseudotherapies and other "remedies" used today for almost any disease? An interesting surgical placebo effect was reported only recently: The ligation of the mammary arteries was considered effective surgery in the treatment of angina pectoris, but this operation proved to be an unsound and dangerous one. The mere exposure of the arteries without ligation and the patient's being handled pre- and postoperatively with the same grave concern shown when the "real" operation was performed was found to be equally effective, so that the very real relief was simply a placebo effect (Beecher 1961). Sham electro-convulsive therapy has been used effectively in psychiatry, and Forrer (1964) remarked that not uncommonly, a patient, mistaking out of ignorance a diagnostic procedure for a therapeutic one, expresses satisfaction with what is erroneously taken to be treatment. Some patients will thank the white-bedecked technician, mistaken for a physician, for the wonderful relief they have just experienced from severe headache, when in actuality the "treatment" was nothing more than the routine performance of an EEG. These modern-day treatments are admittedly less bizarre than the ancient ones mentioned above, but their modus operandi is probably not much different.

While the literature on the history of medicine per se has given due credit to the practices and discoveries of the non-Western world, the literature on the history of the placebo effect has not. Few writers in this area have had anything at all to say about the medicine of the Orient, Africa, Mexico, or Peru, so brief mention will be made of a few aspects of healing in some of these areas in ancient times. The history of sub-Saharan Africa is largely undocumented. Apart from archeological findings, we know little of practices in early African medicine. The assumption that current witchdoctor practices might well be a reflection or relic of ancient ones does not hold when one takes the massive changes in tribal cultures and migrations into account. However, what Schimlek (1950) called the "magic control of chance" was probably just as essential a factor in ancient (and much current) African folk medicine as it was anywhere else in primitive medicine, and as it might be even today in some aspects of the placebo effect.

On the Indian subcontinent, the *Susruta Samhita*, published about 500 A.D., contained detailed descriptions, probably the first ever, of couching for cataract. Plastic nasal surgery was also described in this work, which is considered one of the "greats" of ancient Indian medicine (Thornwald 1962). Apparently, ancient Brahminic doctors were more skilled in surgical techniques than in medical ones, although mention of rauwolfia was made in some ancient manuscripts. Its discovery was probably empirical and most other substances used were undoubtedly placebos. (Rauwolfia is a shrub whose dried roots produce an alkaloid used pharmacologically primarily as a hypotensive and sedative). We do not know much about "placebos" used in India, Ceylon, or the Himalayan areas, but in Chinese medicine much use was made of what we would now refer to as inert medication and therapeutics. The conversations of the Yellow Emperor Huang-ti (ca. 2600 B.C.) and his minister Ch'i Po form the basis of the famous *Nei-Ching* (i.e., "The Theory of Internal Diseases"), which is still in use today. Huang-ti introduced into Chinese medicine the principles of the ancient Chinese philosophy of nature, which regarded the human body as an image of the cosmos and health as dependent on the harmonious balance of the *Yin* and the *Yang*. Acupuncture and pulse doctrine, together with the extensive use of the ginseng plant, were the basis of much of this and later Chinese medicine. With the current Sinophile *Zeitgeist,* most people are now aware that in China today, "modern" (i.e., Occidental) academic medicine still walks hand-in-hand with ancient folk medicine, and a doctor practicing there has to be equally familiar with both, including the wealth of practical experience of the latter (acupuncture, the use of herbs, and so forth). Chinese folk medicine is currently the object of much research aimed at assessing both the extent to which it can be considered placebotypic and the ways in which Western medicine can start understanding radically different concepts of disease and treatment. The recent publication of *A Barefoot Doctor's Manual* (1977), translated into English, allows us an excellent opportunity to view the ways in which the "chijiao yisheng," or barefoot doctor, integrates traditional Chinese medicine and Western medicine. In some ways, the system is much like what we have described above about the history of medicine: Whatever works is used, whatever does not work is discarded in a very pragmatic way. In addition, the system provides a nice combination of allopathic and preventive medicine, thereby forcing a reconsideration of an overadherence to a Western paradigm and allowing us to consider carefully statements such as that of Carlson (1975) who wrote that ". . . the practice of [Western] medicine is an alloy of art, hunch, science and a lot of slavish adherence to dogma" (p. 20).

In Japan, too, there was a flourishing medical spirit, but the indigenous medicine of Japan, which was practiced by the priests, was completely displaced by Chinese medicine in the ninth century A.D. (Pollack and Underwood 1968). Many details of the medicine of Assyria and Babylon, that of ancient India, the doctors of ancient China, the medicine of early Mexico and Peru have been given elsewhere and will not be documented here (see Thornwald 1962; Pollack and Underwood 1968). What is of importance is that we do not assume in a chauvinistic way that medicine originated and grew only in the cultures of the Judeo-Christian world.

Whether the view was taken that medicine's role was to conquer diseases caused by evil spirits (which would be expelled by the ingestion of nasty substances; hence the origin of so many medicines based on excrements, and so forth) or by other forces, a huge variety of substances was, as we have noted, used in ancient, medieval, and even recent medical practice. Through the vicissitudes of availability, practice, and custom, some substances were seen to be better remedies than others; "The fact that a given drug remained long in the pharmacopoeia might mean that (like foxglove, the source of digitalis) it had some genuine therapeutic value, though it might merely be a tribute to the power of suggestion" (Hall and Hall 1964, p. 109).

This book is not meant to be a history either of medicine or of the placebo effect, but rather the brief details given above are meant to show that the parallels between what was effective thousands of years ago and what can be effective now, in our age of "scientific enlightenment," are first of all too striking to be dismissed as coincidence and secondly somewhat disquieting unless we bear in mind the fact that medical theory and medical practice must be judged by different standards. In no other way can we resolve the great discrepancy between the status of scientific knowledge and the efficacy of therapeutic practices at any point in medicine's history.

Hippocrates, in the fifth century A.D., called medicine not a science but an art, and successful physicians were until the nineteenth century judged more by their relationship to their patients than by any other standard. Since medical theory is essentially the zoology of *Homo sapiens,* it bears an appreciable relationship to science. At times medical theory outpaced and at other times fell far behind effective therapy in its scientific "truth" and effectiveness. "It is unfortunately true that the best and most ingenious of theories may lead to disastrous practice, and on the contrary a foolish and erroneous theory may conceivably produce quite satisfactory practice" (Hall and Hall 1964, p. 411). Clearly, there is far more to effective therapy than a knowledge of the functional relationships among the factors that can be considered, in a broad sense, to be physical (e.g., pharmacological, surgical). Whenever we are dealing with non-specific factors, we are dealing with psychological ones, and to some degree, we are *always* dealing with nonspecific factors. "Modern medicine no longer relies chiefly upon the placebo effect or the doctor-patient relationship. An increasing number of drugs and medical procedures have been developed that have a high degree of specificity and predictability . . . ; although psychological and emotional factors may be minimized, however, they cannot be excluded (Shapiro 1963, p. 164)." This latter consideration must be appreciated not only when we are concerned with treatment, but also when we are concerned with etiology, even if to a minimal degree: "Actually, the only patient who can present a malady due solely to structural disease is an unconscious patient" (Harrison 1963, p. 4). Since few doctors have been willing to admit this, perhaps an examination of some factors in medical progress will reveal the reasons.

Progress in medicine shifted the focus of treatment from spirits or demons to some vague inkling of natural causes. In this progress, the *aggregate* known as "illness" no longer existed. Rather, physicians spoke of ailments and specific organs and sites, with diagnostic categories being the order of the day. The nineteenth century pathologist Virchow said: "There are no general diseases, only diseases of organs and cells" (Zweig 1966, p. 10). Every illness was now traced to its origin and then assigned to an already outlined and described category. Once this step was accomplished, all that remained was for the doctor to apply the prescribed therapy to the particular case. Sickness was not something that attacked the whole person, but merely an organ, or a few cells. Better microscopes, increased surgical sophistication, better diagnoses—in short, technology—allowed medicine to make massive strides. "Sickness" no longer meant what it had to primitives; it became, not a human being with an illness, but a case of disease "x", of duration "y", with treatment "z". Medicine had moved a long way from the time when Aristophanes considered it to be one of the arts taught to the Greeks by divine poets (Kudlien 1976). But the elements in medicine that constitute "the art of healing" remained, largely in the guise of the placebo effect. Surgery, as distinct from medicine, always had less of an element of placebo. Majno (1975) has given a beautiful exposition of the early history of surgery across many cultures, and this history makes apparent that the placebo effect is perforce not as powerful there, either historically or now. Most of the studies on the placebo effect we shall view here will be in the realm of medicine rather than that of surgery.

The general healing enterprise, which in most of the Western world is thought of largely in terms of medicine and surgery, sometimes seems embarrassed about its forebears. Small wonder then that many people in the healing professions think that perhaps an acknowledgment of the placebo effect will mean a return to the barbershop and the priesthood from which these professions have dragged themselves up. This statement is not a cynical or pejorative one: Shapiro (1960) noted how many physicians consider the placebo effect something that operates more often in the practice of others and less often in their own. (In the past few years I have also frequently noticed the same attitude in physicians with whom I have worked closely in the psychological problems of medical practice.)

The placebo effect in modern medicine is widespread and common. Reports are appearing with increasing frequency in the medical and psychological literature, but not many speculations as to *how* placebos work have been advanced. As has already been mentioned here, placebos are often viewed more as indicators of the ineffectiveness of physical methods of therapy than as indicators of the power of psychological factors. Taking this to its (logical? absurd?) extreme, one writer has even posed the questions, first, of whether any real medicines exist, since inert ones can treat apparently real diseases just as well as active ones, and second, whether "we aren't all false doctors who seem to treat false sicknesses with false medicines" (Meyer-Bisch 1967, p. 138; my translation). The situation is almost as if a two-way mind-body battle were in progress, with the mind being on the winning side—hence the embarrassment, for such mental processes are that much harder to investigate and in this context might even to the more tough-minded smack of the taboo, the bizarre, and therefore the "unscientific." "Man is attracted to the bizarre . . . the fact that he enjoys contact with the unique situation does not at all mean that he wishes to understand it" (Watkins 1963, p. 96). Perhaps those who encounter the placebo effect do not "enjoy" it because of its bizarreness, but what is bizarre today might not be so tomorrow, when it might become understandable in the language of science. This attribute would make it a respectable member of the scientific bloodline, sired by scientific psychology out of medicine, and vouchsafing the pedigree. What is nonspecific today might become "specific" tomorrow, and the placebo effect might no longer so discomfit those who see it in terms of an analogy between active versus inert medications and science versus magic. I do not feel that this is an overstatement of the case. Shapiro has repeatedly pointed out that the placebo was used originally as a pejorative and derisive epithet to describe the treatment of others and was not knowingly or deliberately prescribed by physicians (e.g., Shapiro 1971a). The criterion for placebo treatment is nowadays based on more than mere opinion about what effective treatment is, and should be based on scientific methodology and principles of controlled evaluation.

Chomsky once wrote something on the mind-body problem (admittedly, he was discussing the psychology of language and not writing about placebos at all) that may have a parallel with what we are discussing here. If we substitute "nonspecific" for "mental," "specific" for "physical" in the following quotation, the whole issue might not seem so mysterious after all:

Ultimately, I think that there will definitely some day be a physiological explanation for the mental processes that we are now discovering . . . it seems to me that the whole issue of whether there's a physical basis for mental structures is a rather empty issue, for the simple reason that if you look over the course of the history of modern science, what you discover is that the concept "physical" has been extended step by step to cover anything that we understand . . . when we ultimately begin to understand the properties of mind, we shall simply, I'm sure, extend the notion "physical" to cover these processes as well [Chomsky 1968, p. 691].

We might add to this Fisher's (1970a) words of caution: "It is one thing to demonstrate that non-specific factors may influence drug response. It is a very different thing to conclude that the mechanism for the observed relationship must be equally non-specific in nature" (p. 19). Many doctors consider ailments in which there is a very clear measure of psychological or psychosomatic involvement to be trivial. They are not, of course, trivial to the sufferers, especially when they worsen. It behooves us to find out as much as we can about what nonspecific variables in treatment are and how, when, where, and why they operate.

2

The Physical Characteristics of the Placebo Itself

When one thinks of the word "placebo," one thinks essentially of a situation in which the physician knowingly gives the form but not the substance of treatment. We will try to find out whether the type of placebo administered will significantly affect its efficacy. For example, will the color and size of a large, red, lactose-filled gelatin capsule be the factors that make it work, or are such factors apparently inconsequential, so that we can consider them irrelevant and thus, redirect our focus toward other independent variables? As is to be expected, research on the form (color, shape, size, and so forth) of placebos has been carried out, but the research has, as we shall see, been quite inconclusive.

Let us first consider the theoretical explanations that have been advanced for the operation of the placebo itself. We shall then review and criticize the research and finally, in this chapter, consider how much light the research has shed upon the importance of the physical characteristics of the placebo itself.

Theoretical Explanations

Psychoanalytic Theory

According to Forrer (1964), the genesis of the placebo effect must be sought in infancy. A hungry infant cries whenever what Forrer calls the "hunger tide" is at its flow. If no food is consumed, the hunger tide ebbs and flows, with the sensation of hunger itself diminishing or disappearing, and then returning, in a cyclical manner. If milk is withheld, the infant, having vocalized discomfort, falls asleep, as the cyclic ebb and flow of the hunger tide repeats itself. The experience of the hunger tide and the infant's perception of his or her own cry leads to an association between the cry and the physiological ebb of the hunger tide. "It is as though the primitive logic of the unconscious ignoring, as it invariably does, any considerations of reality, declares 'the pain I felt disappeared because of those auditory stimuli I took in' " (Forrer 1964, p. 658). Forrer equates this process with an hallucination and cites research of his own (Forrer 1960) showing the hallucinations are either abolished or ameliorated as a consequence of incorporated activity on the part of the hallucinator. These incorporative activities need not be confined to eating and drinking, indeed, Forrer claims, sensory experiences in whatever modality frequently produce identical effects because of the psychological significance of "taking in," by the way of the sense organs, stimuli originating outside them. Proceeding from this point, Forrer claims that sensory stimuli and milk can be equated as being efficacious in relieving the feeling of emptiness experienced in the course of the hunger tide. Since, in the unconscious, all perceptual modalities are equated with one another and because they are all receptor organs, all are equated with the mouth that receives the hunger-relieving milk. The perception (i.e., the hallucination) is equated with milk because both (insofar as the unconscious is concerned) relieve the pain of emptiness when incorporated. Thus, the placebo too displaces an hallucination of emptiness, since the placebo is incorporated. "It is not difficult to understand how an orally-administered medicine can come to be equated with the pain-relieving milk of the patient's infancy" (Forrer 1960, p. 660). Anything that enters any portion of the body can become symbolically equated with that first relief that the infant obtained at the breast and at the bottle, and thus an injection can be a placebo too. Since animals have no capacity for symbolization, placebo effects are inoperative as far as they are concerned, according to Forrer. (However, this assertion is not true, since the placebo effect does occur in animals, as we shall see in the next chapter.)

Forrer's theory can be criticized on several fronts. The constructs are vague and are difficult to relate to any external referent, as are the unconscious processes whereby all perceptual processes are equated with one another. To operationalize these is well-nigh impossible: No observations have been carried out in any controlled, systematic way, and the hypotheses of which the constructs form a part are difficult to refute and impossible to test. There is therefore no firm evidence supporting this particular psychoanalytic theory of the placebo, and it leads us no further in understanding whether or not the physical nature of the placebo is of any importance in its operation.

Learning Theory

The two major approaches in learning theory are classical (or respondent or Pavlovian) conditioning and instrumental (or operant or Skinnerian) conditioning. In classical conditioning, an unconditioned stimulus such as food is presented to a subject. The response, salivation, that is elicited is known as the unconditioned response. Now, if another stimulus, such as the sound of a bell, is presented simultaneously with or just after the food, the previously neutral bell may after a number of pairings elicit the response, salivation, when it is presented to the subject without food. The response the bell alone elicits is called a conditioned response. The persistent absence of the unconditioned stimulus (food) will result in a weakening and eventual diminution or cessation of the conditioned response (salivation) in a process known as extinction.

A conditioned response, once acquired, is not solely elicited by stimuli identical to the original stimulus. Other similar stimuli may elicit the response in a process known as generalization. The degree to which the new stimulus is similar to the original stimulus will affect the strength of the response, with the amount of generalization being positively correlated with the similarity of the second stimulus with the original stimulus situation. Discrimination is achieved by selectively reinforcing (i.e., by providing the unconditioned stimulus after a response) and extinguishing certain responses; when one stimulus is selectively reinforced while another is extinguished, the subject learns to respond to the selectively reinforced stimulus and not to the other.

Operant conditioning entails the emission of a response to a situation. This response is followed by the occurrence of an environmental event contingent upon the emitted behavior. This process is known as reinforcement: The reinforcer here is any environmental event that increases the probability that the response will again be emitted in similar situations in the future, and the particular stimulus is known as the reinforcing stimulus. A discriminative stimulus, according to Ullman and Krasner (1969), marks the time or place when an operant response will have reinforcing consequences. In other words, it is the occasion upon which responses are followed by reinforcement.

In Ullman and Krasner's (1969) view, the "placebo serves as a discriminative stimulus because of its previous associations with curative agents. Thus pills that are very large and imply highly potent medication are more effective than medium-sized pills. A hot color is advisable, while a pill that looks like aspirin has one strike against it" (p. 77). Although Ullman and Krasner cite no experimental support for their statement, the scientific elements of learning theory have been firmly enough established for us to consider such explanations useful here. However, in view of the widespread (and effective) use of aspirin, the generalization *decrement* with a large, red, "hot" pill, as opposed to aspirin, might well be considerable, rather than the opposite being the case as Ullman and Krasner maintained. Without an actual experiment hypothesizing "hot" colors to be more effective than those looking like aspirin, such suppositions, no matter how well grounded theoretically, remain just that—suppositions—and not empirical statements. Let us therefore turn to the research literature and see whether we can learn more.

Research on the Physical Characteristics of the Placebo Itself

The Color and Taste of the Placebo

A case report cited by Kissel and Barrucand (1964) described a subject who could not fall asleep unless he took a sleeping tablet or a placebo, both of which had to be yellow; no capsule of any other color had any effect. Is this case an example of a particular patient's eccentricity, or does research point to the effectiveness of particular colors for particular classes of medication?

Kissel and Barrucand, writing of the color of the placebo, suggest that particular attention should be paid to this particular aspect—laxatives, for example, should be brown and should taste salty—and in writing of the taste of placebos, they suggest that hypnotics should be bitter. Several of the writers in this area have commented simultaneously on the color and the taste of the placebo. Kissel and Barrucand (1964) have said that a bitter placebo is generally more effective than a tasteless one, but they cite no research for this. Glaser and Whittow (cited by Honigfeld 1964a) found no differences in incidence of side effects attributed to sweet white placebos versus bitter red ones. Gammer and Allen (1966) found that neither phenobarbital nor lactose placebos affected the reported emotional state of college student subjects, apparently because over 70 percent of them thought they had received placebos and not a drug. The sweet taste experienced when chewing the capsules was apparently very important in contributing to the skepticism, and the authors found that this incredulity was alleviated by using hard tablets instead of capsules, eliminating the lactose base, and coating the placebo with ascorbic acid. According to Forrer's (1964) psychoanalytic theory, which we examined above, the sweet taste of the lactose placebos would, if anything, have been quite close to that of the mother's milk, which the placebo allegedly symbolizes, so that the opposite results should have been obtained. Gowdey, Hamilton, and Philp (1967) reported that subjects given a red and white gelatin capsule containing lactose took considerably longer to perform an arithmetic test after medication then before, as compared to subjects given a green and yellow one. Seventy-five percent of the subjects given the green and yellow capsules reported one or more side effects, and 84 percent of those given the red and white ones reported one or more side effects, but due to the relatively small number of subjects in each group ($n = 12$), these differences were not significant. (Note that in this study, performance differences *were* significantly different for the two groups or controls.) The latter two studies were not, however, carried out on patients, and for various reasons to be discussed later, whether subjects are patients or not is an important distinction to bear in mind.

Lasagna, cited by Honigfeld (1964a), has said that to guard against the possibility that the patient will ask the pharmacist about the contents of the prescription, physicians are well advised to steer clear of milk sugar (another strike against Forrer's psychoanalytic formulation?) or other well-known placebo ingredients. He recommends various "vile-tasting and vividly-colored tinctures which are not only impressive in physical properties but bear names calculated to inspire confidence in the erudition of the prescriber. Names such as ammoniated tincture of valerian can safely be revealed to the patient without upsetting the psychological applecart . . . colorless capsules are presumed to be unimpressive. One writer advises yellow, orange, or brown; another prefers pink, blue or a mottled design . . . tasteless placebos are considered inferior to bitter or flavoured ones. It is believed that an extraordinarily large pill impresses by its size, an exceptionally small one by its 'potency' " (p. 151).

While Ullman and Krasner's view of the placebo as a discriminative stimulus, and in particular their comments on aspirin, would appear to be in agreement with the above views, this literature may be internally inconsistent, since aspirin, the most widely used medication, would probably be the initial stimulus in the generalization gradient, thereby eliciting the strongest response rather than the weakest, as is implied by all the apparent insistence on a rainbow of colors rather than the somewhat mundane appearance of an aspirin tablet. In all likelihood, therefore, the placebo-giving situation, at least as far as tablets or capsules (and for that matter, all oral medicines) are concerned, is a great deal more complex than can be accounted for merely by the physical appearance and taste of the particular placebo being administered, and the discriminative stimulus value lies in the situation rather than merely in the particular placebo being used.

Research on the Power of Parenteral versus Oral Placebos

Lasagna (cited by Honigfeld, 1964a) maintains that "an injection is thought to be more effective than something taken by mouth: presumably the presence of the nurse or physician necessary for the injection is an important part of the psychological effect" (p. 151). Again, little evidence exists to support this view, for not more than about five studies are to be found comparing placebo response to injections versus pill taking. Some reports that merely test the placebo effect of injection, without comparison or control groups, obviously cannot attest to its strength, since, as has already been mentioned, almost any treatment can carry with it at least some placebo effect.

Kissel and Barrucand (1964) cite an experiment by Traut and Passarelli who treated rheumatic patients with regular placebo injections in the deltoid region. They found that when the injections were, to use Kissel and Barrucand's phrase, *in loco dolenti* (at the site of the pain), relief was greater than when given elsewhere. Goldman, Whitton, and Scherer (1965) carried out an experiment on thirty-two chronic male schizophrenics on two separate wards in order to test two hypotheses, one of which was that more reactions (seen as deactivation in behavior) would be produced by a "drug" given parenterally than one adminis-tered orally. This hypothesis was not supported, despite Shaw's statement (cited by Honigfeld 1964a) that because of their psychological effect, injections are probably more potent than pills. Two more contradictory studies were cited by Honigfeld (1964a): Goldman et al. (1963) found that the effect of suggestion on placebo response was no more pronounced under parenteral than oral conditions of administration, while Morison et al. (1961) reported that claims of improve-ment by arthritic patients were significantly greater with parenteral than with oral administration of placebos. Kissel and Barrucand (1964) stated that in giving an injection, what counts above all is the prick of the needle rather than what is in the syringe.

Looking at the experiments mentioned here, I venture a guess that two important subject variables might explain the contradictory experimental results concerning the prick of the needle. First of all, subjects who have received a long series of injections might have become so accustomed to the slight pain involved that they might not bat an eyelid when given yet another one. Presumably, with the rheumatic patients in Traut and Passarelli's experiment, an injection *in loco dolenti* would have been more painful than one given elsewhere, and this factor might account for the lack of accommodation to the pain on their part. Of course, this guess will have to be investigated further. The second subject variable that occurs to me is one that might manifest itself in schizophrenic patients, such as those in the study by Goldman et al. (1965) mentioned above. The marked difference in reactivity to low-intensity pain, which has, according to Maher (1966, p. 337), been found in chronic schizophrenics as compared to nonschizophrenic subjects (chronic schizophrenics hardly feeling any pain at all), might account for the "ineffectiveness" of this type of placebo with these patients if the prick of the needle is indeed what supposedly makes placebo injections effective.

Comments and Conclusions

"Placebo therapy seems to be consistent with the practice of the medieval physician whose concoctions were as foul-smelling and evil-tasting as possible. Apparently, treatment without specific indications should be imbued with a large component of hocus-pocus, and ideally be administered at the cost of some discomfort to the patient" (Honigfeld, 1964a, p. 151). The experimental evidence that the physical characteristics of the placebo may play a role in its effects is rather sparse, and few studies designed to test these factors have been reported. Other "physical" characteristics assumed to be of importance (e.g., Kissel and Barrucand's [1964] statement that the more expensive the placebo, the more effective it will be) have yet to be investigated. Given what little evidence we have (on the basis of experimentation), we cannot, at the present time, draw any conclusions or make any recommendations for treatment. Different experiments have been so heterogeneous in subjects, type of placebo and its administration, and symptoms to be treated that any comparison between them is difficult and probably logically indefensible right now. Clearly, a series of studies relating such physical aspects of treatment as were mentioned above to the therapeutic outcomes in each case is necessary before any further statements on this aspect of the placebo can be made. Furthermore, in such studies the nature of the subjects and their symptoms should be quite clearly stated, and care should also be taken in assessing the familiarity the subjects have with the particular mode of treatment. Until more carefully designed and executed studies are presented, statements on desirable physical characteristics of placebos intended for specific patient groups will have to remain a matter of intuition, and unfortunately, intuition *is* largely a matter of hocus-pocus. Thus, in looking back to Ellenberger's (1970) comments in the introduction, one is forced to wonder whether his claim that "in scientific therapy there is a dichotomy between physical and psychic therapy" is really so. And in the meantime, we must look elsewhere for the modus operandi of the placebo.

Since the nature of the placebo itself (whether pill or capsule or blue or green or yellow or pink or fluid or injection) does not appear to be the prime determinant of the placebo effect, we must expand our search into other aspects of situations in which placebos are administered. What might some of these be? We shall examine studies and theoretical perspectives covering such diverse aspects of the problem as who gives the placebo to whom, under which circumstances and for which complaints. We shall begin by examining animal studies of the placebo effect and then turn to research on human subjects who are not patients.

3

The Laboratory Study of the Placebo Effect in Nonpatient Subjects and Placebos and Analgesia

The Classical Conditioning Perspective

Animal Studies

Obviously, animals cannot tell us in any direct way about the subjective effects of any psychopharmacological manipulation. The three studies that will be examined here were undertaken as attempts to demonstrate the usefulness of various theoretical formulations as possible explanatory models for the placebo effect in humans, with particular attention being focused on aspects of the classical conditioning model.

Herrnstein (1962) views the placebo effect in terms of Pavlovian conditioning: "The elicitation of a specific reaction by arbitrary agents, such as the abatement of a symptom after the mere sight of a physician and his medicines, may be nothing more than simple conditioning of the sort originally demonstrated by Pavlov with animals" (p. 677). Herrnstein conducted an experiment that attempted to obtain a placebo effect by simulating the known effect of scopolamine on the learned behavior of rats. Scopolamine depresses responding on an intermittent reinforcement schedule, and rats injected peritoneally with scopolamine showed typical scopolamine effects. The experiment demonstrated that an injection of saline could come to depress the responding of a rat that had occasionally been given scopolamine. Herrnstein said that this depression of responding can be termed a placebo effect and that the characteristics of the depression and the way in which it was elicited suggest that it is an example of Pavlovian conditioning. "It seems probable that the CS includes the injection of a hypodermic needle into the peritoneal cavity, for mere handling of the animal in several 'mock' injections did not result in any noticeable change in responding" (p. 678). This placebo effect was based on the animal's experience and could be eliminated by withholding the drug in conformity with the paradigm of simple Pavlovian conditioning. Herrnstein suggests that there appears to be no reason to suppose that the placebo effect in human patients differs in any way, other than in the degree of complexity, from the effect demonstrated in the experiment and that the complexity can be understood as instances of stimulus and response generalization gradients.

That Herrnstein was understating the complexity of the problem can be appreciated if we consider the results of an experiment conducted by three researchers at the German Academy of Science, Berlin. Hecht, Hecht, and

17

Treptow (1968) conducted an experiment to examine the relationships between the functional state of the central nervous system (CNS) and the "conditioned pharmacological effect" (placebo effect) in male albino rats. Benactyzine (7.5 mg/kg) and ethyl crotyl barbiturate (20 mg/kg) affected the conditioned escape response in different ways, depending on the intensity of illumination (0.2 to 0.5, 15 and 1,000 meter-candles). Benactyzine increased the length of the reaction time of the escape response (the darker the illumination, the longer the RT), while ethyl crotyl barbiturate decreased the number of successful escape responses (the darker the illumination, the fewer successful escape responses), as compared to controls. Substitution of sodium chloride solution after ten to twelve trials produced the same response rates, with the conditioned responses changing quantitatively and qualitatively in relation to the intensity of illumination, just as they had done with the active drugs. These results would seem to indicate that the placebo effect is understandable in terms of classical conditioning, with different extero- and interoceptive environmental circumstances affecting the CNS and leading to clearly different placebo effects. The design of this experiment was rather more complex than that of Herrnstein (1962) described above in that it takes environmental changes into account. Unlike Herrnstein, however, Hecht et al. state quite explicitly their reluctance to extrapolate their findings to humans, thereby making clear that such extrapolations must only be made with great caution.

Another experimental study using rats was conducted by Pihl and Altman (1971). After measuring a base level of activity, they measured the drug effects of 3 mg/kg of the stimulant d-amphetamine sulphate solution (AMP) administered interperitoneally. These researchers found that, when different groups of eight rats each were measured after three, nine, or fifteen pairings of drug and trial, activity levels increased. Then the placebo (saline solution) was administered. The groups differed significantly from each other, with the number of pairings between the injection of the drug and placement in the experimental chamber differentially affecting the placebo response. For three pairings of drug and experimental chamber, one out of eight rats (12.25 percent) showed a placebo response. For nine pairings, six rats out of eight (75 percent) showed a placebo response, and for fifteen pairings, all rats (100 percent) showed a placebo response. When continually run under placebo conditions, six of the eight rats in the fifteen-pairing group continued to show a high increase in activity to the saline injection after twenty extinction trials.

A control study was successfully run to rule out the possibility that the higher activity scores of the placebo phase were a function of the residual effects of the daily injections of AMP or the physical effects from the large number of interperitoneal injections. When the tranquilizer chlorpromazine (3 mg/kg interperitoneal chlorpromazine) was substituted for the AMP and the same procedure was used, a significant reduction in activity occurred in the drug phase, but no placebo response was shown when the saline solution was substituted. Activity rebounded from the low drug scores to levels significantly greater than the preceding baseline. According to the authors, the applicability of the conditioning model to the placebo effect may be related to the nature of the active substance used, with a probable interaction between the applicability of the conditioning model, the nature of the active substance, and the form of the response to be measured.

Pihl and Altman note that contrary to the traditional conditioning paradigm, explicitly stating what the conditioned stimuli were in their study is quite difficult: "possible conditioned stimuli are (1) the experimental chamber and the many stimuli associated with it, (2) the procedure of injection used in giving the original drug and/or (3) the presence of the injected material in the body cavity . . . work in defining the conditioned stimuli and the effect of conditioning histories is required, as it may be quite relevant to the human placebo phenomenon" (p. 94).

Although, as Barber and Silver (1968a; 1968b) have argued, experimenter bias might not be as pervasive a phenomenon as fashion might lead one to believe, the fact that it might well still be operative would make a strong case for the inclusion of double-blind precautions in the experiments reviewed above. The double-blind method, which prevents either the subject or the experimenter from knowing when either the active drug or placebos are being given, cannot be disregarded *even in experiments in which the subjects are animals.*

The above studies made some attempt to explain the placebo effect in terms of well-known psychological constructs of greater utility than the rather molar but often-advanced concept of "suggestibility"; both the Hecht et al. study and that of Pihl and Altman attempted to relate the *complexity* of the placebo situation in human beings to more complex experimental analogues than that used by Herrnstein. The former two studies might offer lines of research worth pursuing, but again we encounter the difficulty of using laboratory analogues (let alone animal subjects), which is so confounding here, and we would do well to heed the warnings of Hecht et al. in relation to extrapolating the findings of these studies to the human situation. Let us therefore examine an experiment conducted along essentially the same lines as the ones above, but with human subjects.

A Human Study Based on the Classical
Conditioning Perspective

In the preceding section, we reviewed several experiments that viewed the placebo effect in animals as a conditioned response, based on the Pavlovian paradigm. An experiment aimed at showing the efficacy of the same paradigm for human subjects was conducted by Lang and Rand (1969). These researchers found that when an antianginal drug, "Anginine" (gliceryl trinitrate), was taken sublingually, increases in heart rate of fifteen beats per minute or more occurred in three out of eight healthy, young female subjects. An identical-appearing and -tasting placebo was substituted in a double-blind procedure. Tachycardia again occurred, but the increase in heart rate was less than that produced by the drug, while headache and palpitations occurred only occasionally. These effects were interpreted as conditioned responses: The active tablet served as the unconditioned stimulus by first eliciting a response and the placebo then became the conditioned stimulus. In view of the small number of subjects in the experiment, and the even smaller number exhibiting a placebo response, one has to accept these findings with some caution. In addition, as tempting as simply accepting Lang and Rand's interpretation of their findings might seem, we have noted that even in the animal experiments the placebo situation was viewed as being very complex. As we shall see through the course of this book, a host of other factors might also be responsible for the placebo effect, and while the most parsimonious explanation is desirable, it should not be emphasized to the neglect of other important factors.

Effects of Placebos on Various Tasks in the Psychology Laboratory

The experiment by Gowdey, Hamilton, and Philp (1967) was mentioned briefly above in connection with the research on the physical characteristics of placebos. Some of its other aspects will be examined here. Twelve groups of four medical students each participated: One student in each group was the "recorder"; each of the other three (volunteers) were randomly assigned to one of two treatment conditions, both of which used placebo capsules (in treatment group A, a green and yellow gelatin capsule filled with lactose and in treatment group B, a red and white gelatin capsule containing lactose), or to a control (a drink of water). Subjects were given several tests of psychomotor and mental performance (e.g., an addition test, a tracking test, and a tremor test), administered before the ingestion of the placebos and repeated at thirty and at sixty minutes thereafter. No large changes in performance occurred, and no evidence of fatigue or facilitation of learning was noted, although the subjects in group B took significantly longer to perform the arithmetic test after medication than before. Toward the end of the experiment, subjects were instructed to check any of twenty-nine listed side effects that they experienced. A total of forty-four side effects was reported: Eight of the twelve in group A and ten of the twelve in group B checked·one or more symptoms. On the day after the experiment, the subjects were debriefed and told that both "treatments" were placebos and not in fact the drug acting on the CNS, which they had previously been led to believe. Many of them were shaken and several volunteered that they would "never forget that experiment" (Gowdey, Hamilton, and Philp, 1967, p.

1321), while at least one did not believe that placebos had been used and said that there must have been some mistake. The authors noted that this experiment probably served as a powerful example of what placebos can do for subjects who would in the future administer them. An interesting question, had the subjects volunteered side effects rather than used the checklist, is whether there would still have been no difference between the two groups in the reported incidence of side effects.

Performance on a dynamometer pull-task was found by Pomeranz and Krasner (1969) to be affected by the administration of a placebo, a salve concocted from neobase and red food coloring and administered to the subjects from a medicinal jar. Control subjects rested for a time equivalent to the length of time required to administer the "drug" to the placebo group. Performance on the dynamometer pull-task was measured before and after the treatment for each group, and the results clearly demonstrated that the procedure used in the experimental group served as a placebo in that subjects, informed that this "drug" would relieve muscular fatigue, performed better than the subjects in the control group.

The effects of meprobamate and placebos on the psychomotor behavior of a group of soldiers were studied by Claridge (1961). Half of the subjects received meprobamate tablets; the other half, identical-appearing inert placebos. Subjects were then asked to report subjective effects, and a large number of those given placebos reported nocebo effects, especially drowsiness and nausea. Performance on a serial reaction-time task was measured continuously for ten minutes, and no significant difference was found between the two groups. Surprisingly, both treatment groups performed well below the level of a comparable group of subjects who did the task under the same conditions except that they had received no pills at all. "Just taking pills was sufficient to depress performance significantly. It is also interesting that the overall effect of the placebos was to slow down, rather than speed up, performance. Although none of the subjects was told what to expect, most of them clearly associated drug-taking with 'being drugged' or being made less efficient in some way" (Claridge 1972, p. 27).

Lehmann and Knight (1960) tested twenty-four healthy female subjects before and after a placebo administered as part of a larger drug study. Twelve psychophysiological and psychometric tests were used. The tests of primarily basic psychological functions—and, consequently also, those most devoid of meaning—were found to be the most placebo-proof. These tests, characterized by a low level of functional integration, were flicker fusion, after-image, tapping, RT, and hand steadiness. More complex tests showed that speed components (e.g., cancellation time, track tracer time) were more placebo-prone, while accuracy components (e.g., cancellation accuracy, track tracer accuracy) were more placebo-resistant. The placebo-proneness of a psychological function, as distinguished from the relative proneness of different persons, was emphasized. Some autonomic nervous system reactions and psychological functions requiring considerable integration (e.g., motivational factors, emotional reactions, personal aspects of painful experiences) appeared to be placebo-prone. Placebo-resistant functions included more fundamental psychological processes requiring a minimum of integration.

The studies that have been mentioned here have been quite heterogeneous, so a summary by way of comparing them is difficult. For one thing, the instructions that subjects were or were not given differed considerably from study to study, and as will be shown in a later section of this book, such instructions can be important contributors to any observed placebo effect. One methodological point that should be noted here, however, is that when symptom checklists are used, they should ideally be administered both before and after placebo treatment so that changes in the symptoms checked can with assurance be attributed to the placebos and not to other factors that might have occurred in, or outside of, the experimental situation.

Hallucinogenic Drugs and the Placebo Effect

The current interest in the uses and abuses of hallucinogenic drugs has led to a vast amount of experimentation on various aspects of their effects. Barber (1970) noted that more than 2,000 studies concerning the pharmacological, psychological, and therapeutic effects of LSD alone were published between 1943 and 1963. The relationship between such drugs and what happens when placebos are administered in their place makes for interesting reading and points out some thought-provoking results for those who enjoy the various types of intoxication produced by LSD, marijuana, and other hallucinogens. A strong case could be made here for stating that the psychotomimetic effects of some hallucinogenic drugs can be so unpleasant that we should speak of "nocebos" rather than "placebos." However, since not all users do, in fact, react with noxious side affects, we should guard against using the word "nocebo" in all cases. The studies to be reviewed here deal with lysergic acid diethylamide (LSD-25) and also with marijuana.

Lysergic Acid Diethylamide (LSD-25)

Abramson, Jarvik, Levine, Kaufman, and Hirsch (1955) studied responses given to a questionnaire by thirty-three subjects, who were paid, adult volunteers, healthy and nonpsychotic, and expecting to receive a dose of LSD-25. The placebo consisted of 75cc of tap water. The questionnaire used to assess the responses to the placebo inquired about the subjects' physiological and perceptual states. The questionnaire responses were analyzed with a number of other variables (e.g., body weight, scores on the WAIS, and Rorschach test responses).

On the basis of subjects' periodic responses to the questionnaire, and a comparison of these responses with other variables, the subjects were found to react with varying degrees of severity to the placebo. Some subjects gave no positive response to any question, while one gave positive responses to as many as fifteen different questions out of a possible forty-seven during the three time intervals when the questionnaires were administered. About 60 percent responded positively to "Are your palms moist?"; 50 percent, to "Does your head ache?" "Do you feel fatigued?" and "Do you feel drowsy?"; 25 percent, to "Do you feel as if in a dream?" and "Do you feel weak?" Such questions as "Are things moving around you?" and "Do you see double?" received positive ratings from only about 5 percent of the subjects. The symptoms present in 25 percent to 60 percent of the subjects corresponded in general, according to the authors, to certain of the symptoms of the LSD-25 reaction. The greatest number of positive responses was given by most subjects within thirty minutes after the ingestion of the placebo, with the effect tapering off over the next few hours. Other findings of this study will be reviewed in the section of this book dealing with the personality of the placebo reactor.

Barber (1970) mentioned a study by Zegans, Pollard, and Brown (1967), in which graduate students were given either a placebo or a small (0.5 mg/kg) dose of LSD-25. Subjects receiving LSD did not, overall, differ significantly from those receiving placebo in performance on a battery of creativity tests that included remote associations, originality of word associations, and creation of original designs from tiles. This experiment was conducted primarily to assess the effects of LSD-25 on creativity. The fact that nothing happened that could answer the experimenters' questions might be due to two factors. First, because the effects of LSD-25 are such that most psychomotor and intellectual performance is affected adversely by it, tests of such functions given while the drug is still active do not allow subjects the maximum possible utilization and organization of their creative efforts. Second, the type of subject is important, since poets, painters, or musicians might possibly have creative abilities that are quite different from those of nonartistic subjects. When assessing the creativity-enhancing aspects of the drug, then, we need to look carefully at what type of creativity is being measured and how it can, or cannot, be enhanced in this way.

Linton and Langs (1962) gathered data from a placebo group by means of a seventy-five-item questionnaire developed to monitor LSD-25 and placebo reactions. The subjects were male professional actors; thirty were given LSD-25, and twenty were given a tap-water placebo. The questionnaire successfully differentiated placebo and drug subjects both qualitatively and quantitatively. The authors viewed the placebo response as a reaction to a specific situation (shown, in part, by the differences from pretest behavior). The somatic, affective, and limited cognitive changes that occurred were shown in three patterns: (1) succumbing to the situation; (2) becoming bored and hostile; and (3) hardly reacting at all. Different aspects of the placebo response were more prominent at different times, with somatic symptoms and feelings of loss of control being strongest at thirty minutes after ingestion and then declining steadily. After two hours, subjects reported feelings of having acquired new meanings and a more prominent general feeling of disinhibition. The latter persisted through five hours and dropped off by eight hours. Difficulty in thinking reached its maximum at five hours, accompanied by some feelings of things having lost meaning and feelings of elation or silliness. Loss of sense of time, feelings of being inhibited and slowed down, angry or annoyed, and depressed increased steadily and reached their maximum at the end of the day. The authors noted that this sequence was similar to that seen in the LSD-25 subjects, although at a much lower level. The authors found that at two, five, and eight hours after ingestion of the placebo, subjects were individually consistent in their reactions, with some reacting generally strongly and others only weakly. These relationships enabled the authors "to speak of subjects as being 'placebo reactors' or not, within the framework of the experimental day, although we have no evidence on the question of whether these subjects would react similarly in a different experimental setting" (p. 375). The significant personality differences found between strong and weak placebo reactors in this study will be discussed in the section of this book dealing with the personality of the placebo reactor.

The reader will notice, almost consistently in this book, that placebo experiments using nonpatient subjects are criticized on the basis of their low ecological validity. This complaint cannot, however, be justifiably made here, because nonpatient subjects are, when one considers the problem, the ones who usually use hallucinogenic drugs. Another look at the experiments mentioned above will reveal that the milieu in which they were conducted was, however, very different from that in which "acid trips" are usually taken. The ecological validity of the experiments was, therefore, low in that respect, and accordingly, seeing what the effects of "LSD-25" placebos in a situation more akin to the usual one would be is an interesting area for more research. We often consider the laboratory situation to be laden with demand characteristics, but a roomful of "acid freaks" would probably engender even more demand characteristics. Research might also be undertaken on the use of such placebos in medical situations where LSD-25 is administered psychiatrically; for example, the current interest in easing the suffering of dying patients by treating them with it (e.g., Avorn 1973). The effects of placebos substituted for LSD-25 are so striking that the results in real-life situations might be even more interesting and thought provoking.

Marijuana

Marijuana is one of the most widely used psychedelic drugs in the world. The female hemp plant, *Cannabis sativa,* produces a resin, cannabis, which is found in fairly low concentrations in drugs known as *kif* in Morocco, *dagga* in South Africa, *bhang* in India, and marijuana, or more commonly, *grass,* in the United States. The tetrahydrocannabinols are the most active compounds in the cannabis resin, and they produce the commonly known psychological effects of "getting stoned." This compound is usually abbreviated THC.

Hochman and Brill (1971) tested twenty volunteer regular users of cannabis with each of five preparations of marijuana varying in strength from 0 (ether-extracted placebo) to 7.5 mg content of THC. All the subjects had been using marijuana almost daily for three or more years. The samples were smoked through a glass tube, in one end of which the cigarette was placed and from the other end of which the smoke was inhaled. After twenty inhalations on a fixed time schedule, subjects were asked to estimate their level of intoxication after fifteen minutes and again after forty-five minutes. A scale of 0 to 10 was used with 10 being the highest possible level of intoxication in their experience. The researchers found that the greatest intoxication was to the most potent material (7.5 mg THC per cigarette), but, interestingly, chronic users experienced a higher degree of subjective intoxication from the placebo than from low-potency marijuana or placebo plus red oil extract (which had a potency of 5 mg THC per cigarette). Comparison of the mean scores of the different test groups suggested that the psychological factor in intoxication may have exceeded the pharmacological factor until a consumed dose level of 5 mg was exceeded.

Hochman and Brill's experiment is the only one I have been able to locate in which a placebo was used in place of a "joint." Like the LSD-25 experiments, the milieu was not the same as that in which marijuana is commonly smoked. If further research replicates these results, habitual users of such drugs will have a number of points to ponder.

We have examined a number of laboratory studies using nonpatient subjects and have found some evidence that placebos do have effects even when the subjects are not patients. However, drugs and placebos are usually administered only when something goes awry; for example, to provide relief from pain. In the next section we shall examine how placebos affect the experience of pain. The study of pain is an interesting stepping stone between laboratory situations and studies that are purely clinical in nature, since pain can be inflicted in the laboratory and can thus bring us a step closer to clinical situations in which suffering is "real" and does not have to be pretended or imagined. As we proceed, we shall encounter more and more variables that are of extreme importance in "real-life" clinical situations. These variables were not present in the above-mentioned studies, and they are so intimately related to the modus operandi of the placebo effect that we can ill-afford to neglect them, even at the cost of ideally parsimonious experimentation.

Pain, Placebos, and Placebo Analgesia

When the famous poet, John Dryden (1631-1700) wrote "For all the happiness mankind can gain, Is not in pleasure but in rest from pain," he was expressing succinctly and well the feelings that people have about pain and the experience of pain. Although the properties of such analgesics as opium have been known for thousands of years, indeed before the earliest medical records (Eddy and May 1973), not surprisingly, what are considered two of the greatest pharmacological advances of the nineteenth century were the discovery of the alkaloid, morphine, derived from opium and the first use of ether and chloroform as anesthetic agents (Bergersen and Krug 1969). At the turn of the twentieth century, aspirin was first made in Germany. Surgical and other pain, both severe and minor, were thus readily amenable to relief, and pain, though still an extremely common and often severe a phenomenon, became far less terrifying and debilitating an experience for so many of its sufferers. Advances in pharmacological research are increasing the physician's ability to relieve this suffering: The search for better analgesics continues, and solutions for such problems as morphine-type drug dependence, an unfortunate side effect of long-term analgesic administration, are emerging (Eddy and May 1973). Analgesic drugs are routinely evaluated by using the double-blind procedure, with placebos used as the control group. But what of the placebo itself as an analgesic?

Placebos are a form of potent therapeutic intervention in their own right; they can be conceived of as "another active pharmacological agent whose positive analgesic effects can be independently evaluated using the same stringent methods that would be used to test any other potent analgesic agent" (Evans 1974, p. 289). In this section, we shall mention some psychological aspects of pain, consider some qualities of analgesics, and review some studies of placebo analgesia in both experimental and clinical pain. Mention will be made several times of the work of Evans, in particular his 1974 paper on the placebo effect in pain reduction, which, apart from the work of Beecher, is amongst the most outstanding published to date in an area where there is a need for a great deal of further research.

The psychology of pain is an exceptionally complex and often seemingly mysterious area that is being studied with increasing intensity and consequent clarification of many issues and problems. Pain is not, especially in humans, simply a function of the amount of bodily damage. Indeed, as Melzack (1973) has so clearly pointed out in *The Puzzle of Pain,* a number of factors, such as the meaning of the pain, previous painful experiences and our memory of them, and the culture in which we have been brought up, all play an essential role in how we feel pain and respond to it. Taking up the last point, first, we know how childbirth, for example, is conventionally considered in Western culture to be just about the worst pain a person can experience. Yet throughout the world there are cultures in which women interrupt their work in the fields and, almost literally, give birth while squatting in a ditch and then return to the fields after a few hours. An interesting comparison can be made of this practice, known as *couvade,* and the Western practice of turning the delivering mother into a hospital patient, particularly in the United States where childbirth at home, with the assistance of a registered midwife, is virtually unknown. (Even the roles of husbands are different: The husband of the women in *couvade* gets into bed and groans as though he were in great pain while his wife bears the child; the husband of the woman in the delivery room traditionally paces the floor of the waiting area and consumes large amounts of coffee and many cigarettes!) Clearly, the impact that cultural values exercise on the amount of pain experienced during childbirth is enormous.

The fact that the meaning attached to the painful stimulus affects response to pain can also be seen in other situations. For example, Beecher (1959) observed that not more than about a third of soldiers severely wounded in various battles in the Second World War complained of enough pain to require morphine when they were carried into combat hospitals. After the war, however, when Beecher asked a group of civilians who had similar but surgically induced wounds whether they wanted morphine to alleviate their pain, 80 percent claimed pain severe enough to request morphine. Beecher noted that whereas to the wounded soldier the response to the injury experience was relief and thankfulness at escaping alive from the battlefield, to the civilian, undergoing surgery was a depressing, calamitous experience. One can think of many other examples in which the meaning of an apparently identical pain-causing stimulus can result in remarkably different effects ranging all the way from the difference in a child's reactions to a playful slap from a friend and a punishing one from a parent, to the complexities of sexual masochism.

Attention, anxiety, and suggestion are other factors that can contribute to the intensity of the pain experience. All of the above factors will affect pain perception threshold (the lowest stimulus value at which a person reports feeling pain). This observation is an interesting one, since other evidence indicates that all people, regardless of cultural background, have a uniform sensation threshold (the lowest stimulus value at which sensation is first reported; see Melzack 1973). However, such uniformity in sensation threshold is found only in precisely controlled laboratory experiments where all environmental conditions are kept constant and not in nonlaboratory situations. Even more interesting is the effect of cultural factors on pain tolerance levels, where pain and its expression are markedly different.

Melzack and Torgerson (1971) have shown how words descriptive of pain can range in scale value from "mild" to "excruciating" in terms of sensory qualities, affective qualities, and evaluative qualities, and they classified 102 words in this way. Pain is therefore an extremely complex perceptual experience that cannot be defined easily. It is "not a single quality of experience that can be specified in terms of defined stimulus conditions . . . it represents a category of experiences, signifying a multitude of different, unique events having different causes, and characterized by different qualities varying along a number of sensory and affective dimensions" (Melzack 1973, pp. 45-46). What are the qualities of the drugs with which this complex phenomenon is treated?

Bergersen and Krug (1969) have listed the following as the required qualities of an analgesic drug: (1) it should be potent enough to afford maximum relief of pain; (2) it should be physiologically nonaddicting; (3) it should exhibit a minimum of side effects; (4) it should not cause tolerance to develop; (5) it should act promptly and over a long period of time with a minimum of sedation, so that the patient is able to remain awake and responsive; and (6) it should be relatively inexpensive. "Needless to say, no present-day analgesic has all of these qualifications, and so the search for one continues" (Bergersen and Krug 1969, p. 202). The first and fifth qualities, if fulfilled by a placebo, would make it the ideal analgesic, since, with inert placebos in particular, conditions 2, 3, 4, and 6 would apply. Let us examine some of the evidence available on the placebo as an analgesic. We shall discuss placebo analgesia in both experimental and clinical pain.

Placebo Analgesia in Experimental Pain

As Evans (1974) noted, Beecher (1959) found that in experimental studies placebos reduced pain in only 3 percent of the subjects, a much lower figure than in clinical pain. Since Beecher's review, eleven other studies of experimental pain have yielded an average placebo relief of about 16 percent. This improvement "is primarily a result of replacing the once popular radiant heat and electric shock methods of inducing pain with techniques which induce longer-lasting, slow-acting pain, such as the cold pressor and ischemic muscle pain methods" (Evans 1974, p. 290).

A study by Clark (1967) indicates that when rating responses to radiant heat stimuli were obtained from subjects under placebo and control conditions, sensitivity to thermal stimulation remained unaltered, and the sole effect of the placebo was to raise subjects' criterion for pain. Another study by Clark (1969) concerned the administration of a placebo described as a potent analgesic to healthy, paid volunteers. This placebo sharply reduced the proportion of pain responses to radiant heat stimulation, thereby suggesting that the threshold for pain had been raised. However, analysis of the data by sensory-decision theory demonstrated that thermal sensitivity remained unchanged and that the effect of the placebo was solely to alter the subjects' bias or likelihood ratio criterion.

Gelfand, Gelfand, and Rardin (1965) subjected nonpatient subjects to ultrasonic stimulation and administered inert placebos. Subjects were then again exposed to ultrasonic stimulation. The induced thresholds and tolerance of the pain were measured in both administrations. Scores of religiosity and social desirability were significantly positively related to pain tolerance in placebo reactors, but no personality variable was related to pain threshold scores. The hypothesis that pain threshold is more highly loaded with physiological than psychological components, and the reverse for pain tolerance, was supported by the personality relationship found.

Sternbach (1968) has noted: "Two themes occur repeatedly in studies of pain relief by hypnosis and placebos. One is that anxiety reduction and pain relief are associated; the other is that neither procedure is particularly effective in producing pain relief if anxiety is not present in some minimal amount, or if anxiety is kept high by other factors" (p. 145). The variability in the results of the above experiments, and the low percentage of subjects who experience placebo analgesia in experimental, nonclinical studies, might well reflect the absence of any anxiety-inducing experimental manipulation, and as Chapman and Feather (1973) have shown, oral administration of 10 mg diazepam, though not itself an analgesic but rather an antianxiety agent, increases the tolerance to continuing experimental pain and tends to reduce the transitory anxiety associated with the pain experience. Diazepam does not affect the sensory-discriminative aspect of the pain experience, but it does affect the motivational-emotive aspects and in so doing reduces the aversive drive associated with continuing pain.

The close relationship of anxiety levels and pain perception is not well understood. If the administration of a placebo leads to a decrease in anxiety, then Sternbach's comment cited above would suggest that a decrease in the perception of pain would occur. Thorn (1962) has provided some evidence that highly anxious subjects are consistent placebo reactors (in a study that will be examined later in this book in the chapter on the personality of the placebo reactor). When we talk of anxiety, though, we should be aware of the difference between trait anxiety and state anxiety. Trait anxiety is a stable characteristic of the person, whereas transient, situationally determined anxiety can occur in anyone. McGlashan, Evans, and Orne (1969) examined the relationship between placebo analgesia, trait, and state anxiety in a laboratory study on the nature of hypnotic analgesia and placebo response to ischemic muscle pain. Ischemic muscle pain is produced by using a tourniquet to occlude arterial blood flow to the upper arm, which results in a dull aching sensation, the intensity of which increases with increasing ischemia. Unlike electric shock, ischemic pain has some of the qualities of clinical pain, since it is not a transient sensation.

The twenty-four paid, male college volunteers in this study were subjected to ischemic muscle pain in three sessions: (1) baseline pain response testing; (2) after the induction of hypnotic analgesia (for further discussion of which, see both the original 1969 article by McGlashen et al. and the article by Orne 1973), and (3) after the ingestion of a placebo packed in a Darvon Compound-65 capsule. Except for one of the authors, who had no contact with the subjects during this study, all the laboratory personnel were under the impression that half of the capsules contained placebo and half contained Darvon Compound-65, a mild analgesic. All the special advantages of the double-blind method were therefore obtained, without the use of an active drug. The third part of the study is of particular interest here. Thirty-five minutes after the ingestion of the placebo, ischemic muscle pain was administered by having each subject pump a rubber bulb to displace water, while at the same time arterial blood flow was occluded by an inflated sphygmomanometer cuff. Each subject reported the pain threshold (when his arm first hurt or when the sensation became unpleasant) and continued pumping until the pain became intolerably bad and prevented further pumping (pain tolerance). Two measures of anxiety were administered: Generalized trait anxiety was measured by the Taylor Manifest Anxiety Scale, and situation-specific anxiety was measured by the Zuckerman Anxiety Check List. According to Evans (1974), the results indicate quite clearly that the two types of anxiety are independently related to two clearly distinct aspects of the placebo response in this case. Situational anxiety increased after placebo ingestion but, paradoxically, pain tolerance was improved. The increasing levels of situational anxiety correlated only with the increase in the pain threshold, not with pain tolerance. Evans acknowledged that pain thresholds have been notoriously unreliable in that they are prone to the response bias inherent in subjective reports. Since a number of variables extremely prone to response bias and compliance correlated with the pain threshold measures, Evans (1974) noted that "this part of the total response to a placebo medication does not represent any therapeutic factor attributable to the placebo but merely reflects the methodological problems associated with measuring subjective change in cooperative subjects, particularly when they are made temporarily anxious. The non-analgesic effect of placebo is, of course, the factor which the double-blind group was designed to control" (p. 292).

However, placebo-induced changes occurred that were not related to the threshold changes or situational anxiety (or to other measures reflecting response bias). Chronic or trait anxiety was related to improvement in pain tolerance rather than pain threshold. Pain tolerance improved for state anxious subjects and not for nonanxious subjects. This observation is interesting because measures of pain threshold are not of great relevance in situations where "real" clinical pain is much worse than its threshold. Several measures of frequency and intensity of side effects and psychosomatic symptoms reported following placebo ingestion correlated with trait anxiety and pain tolerance, but none correlated with suggestibility or response bias measures, thereby ruling out the responsibility of experimental artifact in these results. So we see that placebos have some of the therapeutic effects of active analgesic agents. Placebo analgesia may be a function of the patient's chronic anxiety level, and as Evans (1974) said, perhaps the patient "can gain control over his tendency to be anxious, which he can temporarily attribute to his pain, by responding to the climate of hope for relief being provided by the 'magic' his physician prescribes, reinforced by the physician's own conviction of the efficacy of his therapeutic intervention" (p. 293). In such situations, placebo effects in trait-anxious people that result in increased pain tolerance may be associated with state anxiety reduction in people who are patients (as opposed to nonpatient subjects).

Placebo Analgesia in Clinical Pain

In a frequently cited work, Beecher (1955) reviewed fifteen clinical studies on the therapeutic effectiveness of placebos in several conditions. Nine of these dealt with analgesia in severe postsurgical wound pain, pain from angina pectoris, and headache. The placebos, route of administration, number of patients, and percentages of satisfactory relief varied. For example, subcutaneous saline for severe postoperative wound pain gave satisfactory relief to 31 percent of the patients; oral lactose relieved 33 percent for the same condition; and 38 received satisfactory relief from angina pectoris pain by taking oral lactose. Satisfactory relief was defined as 50 percent or more relief of pain, in most cases, where pain was rated on a rating scale by the patient. Evans (1974) indicates that subsequent studies confirm Beecher's figures that about a third of patients achieve significant pain relief after ingesting a placebo.

The power of analgesic placebos can be considerable. An analgesic drug that is being evaluated for its relative effectiveness is standardly compared to other analgesics of known effectiveness. The index of drug efficiency obtained (Evans 1974) is expressed by the ratio of the reduction in pain with the unknown active drug, divided by the reduction in pain with the known analgesic. If a mild analgesic such as codeine is compared with morphine, the index would be relatively low, which means that codeine is less effective than morphine. If codeine is compared with aspirin, the index would be greater than 1.00, which shows codeine to be more effective than aspirin. We can perform similar calculations to obtain the index for placebo. Seven studies reviewed by Evans (1974) showed the index of placebo efficiency compared to a standard dose of morphine to be 0.56, thereby indicating placebo to be 56 percent as effective as morphine. (This index is based on the mean reduction in pain for the whole sample, whereas earlier studies based results of the magnitude of placebo effects on the percentage of the sample who subjectively achieved pain reduction of a fixed amount of 50 percent of initial pain. Studies simultaneously comparing several drugs with placebo were excluded.) Based on ten studies (averaged), the index of placebo efficiency for aspirin is not significantly different from that for morphine at 0.54. That for Darvon, an intermediate strength analgesic, is also 0.56. "This is indeed a rather remarkable and unique characteristic for any active pharmaceutical agent! The effectiveness of a placebo compared to a standard dose of a specific analgesic drug administered double-blind is a *constant.* In other words, the effectiveness of the placebo is directly proportional to the apparent effectiveness of the active analgesic agent" (Evans 1974, p. 294). A possibility might be that when a physician is using a powerful analgesic agent such as morphine, double-blind administration produces a strong placebo effect. When a less powerful analgesic such as aspirin is used, the placebo effect is smaller but still proportionately about half as effective as the actual analgesic. Evans maintains that the conviction of the therapist about the drug's potency, which can presumably be communicated to the patient in terms of the plausibility and expectation that it will work, seems to be a powerful mediator of therapeutic effectiveness.

Some General Comments on Placebo Analgesia

The research on placebo analgesia strongly suggests that, at least when working with experimental pain in nonpatient subjects (and to a certain extent with clinical pain, although most clinical research has not included many crucial variables such as anxiety level or satisfactorily distinguished chronic from acute pain), placebos affect pain tolerance but have little or no effect on pain threshold. The distinction between pain sensation and the motivational aspects of pain has been made frequently and was expressed well by Beecher (1959) in terms of the primary and secondary components of the pain experience. The primary component is the pain sensation itself (including the perception, discrimination, and recognition of the noxious stimulus), while the secondary component consists of suffering and reactive aspects (including anxiety and emotional responses to pain). The primary and secondary components are considered to be independent; for example, we have already noted that pain is not a function of the amount of bodily damage alone. With placebo analgesia, we are concerned with the secondary component of the pain experience. Obviously, we are dealing with the influence of psychological processes on pain perception and response. The motivational-affective dimension of the pain experience, covering such aspects as anxiety, attention, and set, can probably influence pain by acting at even the earliest levels of sensory transmission. The degree of control would, however, be partly determined by the temporal-spatial properties of the input patterns. Burn pains, for example, which are almost unbearable in intensity, might rise so rapidly in intensity that the patient is unable to have any control over them, while more slowly rising temporal patterns are susceptible to central control and may allow the use of various psychological stratagems to keep the pain under control.

   Pain therapy can involve manipulating not only the sensory input but also motivational and cognitive factors. We have seen the important role that anxiety plays in placebo analgesia, and we might note with interest that of the psychological approaches for pain relief mentioned by Sternbach (1968), two (desensitization techniques and progressive relaxation methods) are widely used by behavior therapists in anxiety reduction. Possibly, therefore, anxiety reduction is crucial in both pain tolerance and in placebo analgesia. There is still a great deal to be learned about placebo analgesia. As we shall see later on, a host of factors such as patient personality, instructions, therapist personality, and therapist behavior have all been shown to be of importance in the effectiveness of placebos both as antianxiety and other agents. These factors have not been controlled in the studies conducted thus far on placebo analgesia. They should be included in future studies, as should pre- *and* postexperimental measures of anxiety, both trait and state, in order to assess changes in these important variables.

We saw earlier that in studies of experimental pain the average placebo relief has been about 16 percent, while in clinical pain it has been about 33 percent. Some crucial variables must account for the fact that placebos are apparently twice as effective in clinical as in experimental pain. By now we have both theoretical and empirical support for the importance of psychological factors in pain tolerance; might we find some crucial psychological variables in patients that are not found in laboratory situations involving nonpatient subjects? Examination of the literature on the psychology of illness brings out in bold relief how the answer to this question is indeed "Yes." A discussion of some of the aspects of the psychology of illness will be found in the following chapter. This discussion leads quite naturally into the examination of the concept of ecological validity and its great importance (and unfortunate neglect) in most research on the placebo effect.

4

The Psychology of Illness and the Ecological Validity of Placebo Experiments

In the opening sections of this book, we saw how views of illness have changed over the centuries, and an argument for the necessity of considering nonspecific effects in therapy was presented. We have examined various attempts to account for the placebo effect both theoretically and empirically, and the overtures to this chapter have already been sounded in terms of statements indicating that psychological differences between healthy and sick people can be so important that they cannot be neglected when conducting research on the placebo effect. These differences are not merely a matter of intuition about the subject but are borne out by a considerable body of research—much of it quite recent—on the psychology of illness.

The point that illness is not merely a matter of physiological disturbance was forcefully expressed by Jerome Frank (1973) in *Persuasion and Healing*. Frank wrote about the importance of our acknowledging

> . . . that psychological and bodily processes can profoundly affect each other. High among the former are the meanings of illness emerging from the interplay of the sick person with his family and his culture. All illnesses, whatever their bodily components, have implications that may give rise to anxious emotions, raise difficult moral issues, damage the patient's self-esteem, and estrange him from his compatriots. Chronic illness, especially, causes demoralization. Constant misery, forced relinquishment of the activities and roles that supported the patient's self-esteem and gave his life significance, the threat of suffering and death—all may generate feelings of anxiety and despair, which, in turn, may be intensified by reactions of anxiety, impatience and progressive withdrawal in those close to him, especially when his illness threatens their security as well as his own. Thus illness often creates a vicious circle by evoking emotions that aggravate it [pp. 46-47].

What some of these emotions and emotional changes are will now be discussed.

The important distinction between health behavior, illness behavior, and sick-role behavior was made by Kasl and Cobb (1966a, 1966b). Health behavior is any activity that a person who believes himself or herself to be healthy undertakes for the purpose of preventing disease or detecting it while it is still asymptomatic. Illness behavior consists of activities (particularly complaining and consulting other people) undertaken by people when they feel ill in attempts to define their state of health and seek remedy if necessary. Sick-role behavior is shown by people who consider themselves ill and is undertaken in order to become well again. Included here are receiving appropriate treatment and possibly demonstrating several dependent behaviors as well as some degree of neglect of everyday activities. Many changes in behavior, identity, and role performance occur in the various stages in the continuum from health to disease.

In illness behavior there is some degree of psychological distress (predominantly anxiety, depression and its components of resentment, low self-esteem, loss of sense of social support, and guilt and sadness) and the discomfort arising from the symptom. Symptoms may cause psychological distress and vice-versa. Sick-role behavior consists of distress, discomfort, motivation to get well, and performance related to the nature of sick-role norms. Motivation to get well includes personal needs and also environmental and interpersonal incentives and barriers. Sick-role norms include commitment to other social roles, congruence with self-concept, knowledge and internalization of norms, mutuality of doctor-patient expectations, and willingness to conform. Later on in this book we shall see how important the latter two can be in the placebo effect.

Health, illness, and sick-role behavior all have in common the factor of perceived threat of disease and the way that this perception is related to the particular behavior. The most important variable mediating the influence of perceived threat is the perceived value of preventive action, with perceptions of both threat and remedial action being influenced by a number of demographic and background variables. The demands of the sick-role norms are affected by both personality and situational characteristics. Quite clearly, then, we are dealing with a number of important factors that might be quite different in experimental studies, where subjects are not patients, and clinical-type studies, where they are. Beecher (cited by Honigfeld 1964b) interpreted the greater efficacy of placebos in clinical as compared to experimental studies as being due to stress, a factor that potentiates the effectiveness of placebos under clinical conditions. Such stress may be both systemic and psychological, with the latter being the "psychological distress" that is of such importance in illness and sick-role behaviors.

A great deal of research has been conducted in the last few years on both the psychology of health, illness, and sickness and the ways in which stress relates to these states. Although we will not discuss these studies in any detail, some of the noteworthy ones will be reviewed in this section in order to further substantiate the arguments presented earlier regarding the suitability of non-patients as subjects for placebo research. This brief review is, of course, only a very small sample of what is becoming a substantial and influential area of investigation. Lipowski (1969) said that "to understand how the patient experiences his illness and copes with it one has to know what all aspects of his disease mean to him and what responses to his complaints he obtains from other persons, including health professionals. Psychosocial factors influence the course and outcome of every illness, and it is imperative that their evaluation should be a part of medical diagnosis and management" (p. 1197). A volume in *Advances in Psychosomatic Medicine* (Lipowski 1972), dealing with psychosocial aspects of physical illness, includes such contributions as recent life changes and illness susceptibility, the personal meanings of illness, somatic perception during illness, coping with severe illness, and the impact of the hospital environment on the patient. Steinhauer, Muchin, and Rae-Grant (1974) addressed themselves to psychological aspects of chronic illness, including, importantly, not only the effects of chronic illness on the patients (particularly children) but also on their families and those treating them. Mechanic's outstanding work on psychosocial aspects of illness is well known and includes a survey (1972) of some of the literature on social psychological factors affecting the presentation of bodily complaints that shows how a host of nonspecific factors can influence the ways in which people perceive and present what ails them. The comprehensive edited collection of papers on the relationships of stressful life events and physical illness by Dohrenwend and Dohrenwend (1974) includes life change and illness susceptibility, catastrophic illness, and emotional distress. Another recent edited volume (Moos 1977) deals with coping in the face of severe illnesses like cancer, cardiovascular disease, burns, chronic conditions, and organ transplants. In Moos' book we see what sorts of factors are involved in such coping, how severe the stresses can be, and what an enormous disruption can occur from a state of illness and its accompanying psychological processes. Once these works have been read and their implications considered, one is forced to recognize some of the absurdities involved in doing research concerning particular kinds of stressful states (i.e., illness and sickness) on people who are not experiencing such stress. Let us look more closely at some of the aspects of stress that are relevant to this issue.

Selye (1956) sees stress as the state of the organism following failure of the normal homeostatic regulatory mechanisms of adaptation. Selye has been the major worker in research on systemic stress. A major key to the understanding of systemic stress has been the distinction between the specific effects induced by one or another stressor agent and its nonspecific effects. The intensity and duration of both specific and nonspecific effects can produce important changes which, according to Cofer and Appley (1964), "taken together, constitute the sterotypical response pattern of systemic stress . . . [operationally defined by Selye as] a state manifested by a syndrome which consists of all the nonspecifi-cally-induced changes in a biologic system" (p. 442). A large variety of stimulus events (stressor agents), including temperature extremes, infections, hemor-rhage, drugs, injury, surgery and shock, can give rise to such stress. Stressor agents may be both direct (surgical, pharmacological, physical) and indirect (neurogenic or psychogenic). Interestingly and obviously, illness behavior and sick-role behavior may involve both kinds of stressor agents, and when the local or focal adaptation appropriate to the particular form of the stressor are ineffective, or when the stressor is nonspecific, the general adaptation syndrome (GAS) is invoked. The GAS, which consists of three stages (alarm reaction, stage of resistance, stage of exhaustion), involves complex interrelations between neurological, hormonal, and metabolic mechanisms.

Psychological stress is somewhat broader than systemic stress. Appley (cited in Cofer and Appley 1964) proposes that stress is "the state of an organism in any situation where his general well-being is threatened *and* where no readily available response exists for the reduction of the threat (p. 451). A condition of only insufficiency is, however, not enough to produce psychological stress. As Cofer and Appley indicate, the change from innate or habitual to new coping behavior, or the exhaustion of the already existing effective coping responses, permits a change in arousal known as the instigation threshold. If something interferes with goal behaviors, or if such an interference is anticipated, and if this interference continues, then the frustration threshold is reached. Threat is now perceived, anxiety is aroused, and coping behavior is intensified. Exclusively task-oriented, problem-solving behavior is no longer the only behavior, so that ego-oriented self- or integrity-sustaining behaviors arise. Such behaviors would be involved in the "identity" and "behavior" aspects of Kasl and Cobb's (1966a, 1966b) conceptualization of illness behavior and sick-role behavior mentioned earlier. Should task- and ego-oriented behaviors have persisted for a while without any effective change in the situation, the stress threshold is reached. All task-oriented behaviors are eliminated and only ego-protective behaviors remain. Danger may be perceived and possible desperation or panic might occur before the ego-protective behaviors are in turn eliminated, thereby leading to an exhaustion threshold and the perception of helplessness and hopelessness. The latter will not occur in most everyday illnesses, but it is probably what occurs in "giving up the will to live" and in such phenomena as voodoo death (for discussions of which phenomena see Cannon 1957 and Richter 1957).

Psychological stressors may involve either a deficiency or an excess of stimulation as well as ambiguity or conflict of stimuli. When a person is engaged in illness or sick-role behavior, he or she may be removed from the familiar environment, and familiar stimuli may be removed. Cofer and Appley (1964) mentioned these two types of changes as stress-invoking; in addition, the person may be exposed to a large number of both direct and indirect stressor agents, some of which might well be involved in the therapeutic measures that are being undertaken. The person's ability to rely on habitual behaviors is disturbed and he or she moves "up the stress ladder" (Cofer and Appley 1964, p. 455) in order to protect his or her orientation, stability, or integrity. Ambiguity is a stressor because the person cannot know what response is required. Conflict is a stressor because the person is required to perform incompatible responses. Both result in uncertainty, restrictions of response repertoire, and, if unabated, stress. In illness behavior, ambiguity may, for example, arise from a lack of information as to the nature, course, and prognosis of the illness. These are only some of the stressors involved in illness; other factors involved in illness, such as vulnerability, will also increase stress. These factors will seldom be present or if present will not be of the same magnitude in healthy people as opposed to persons who are in a clinical situation for one reason or another or are engaging in illness behavior or sickness behavior. The reasons why aspects of stress and illness must be considered when studying the placebo effect will become even more evident in the following discussion of ecological validity.

In studying a complex phenomenon like the placebo effect, one might hope that using an experimental analogue would provide the ideal research conditions. Cowen (1961) indicates that more rigorous control of extraneous variables, greater refinement of experimental design, and greater depth and precision of measurement of relevant critical functions are the major potential contributions of the experimental analogue method. Maher (1966) notes that "in its simplest form the experimental analogue involves the creation under controlled conditions of an event which is similar to a naturally occurring phenomenon, where our ultimate interest is the phenomenon itself" (p. 105) and states that the term experimental analogue is used "to indicate that we are studying phenomena which are deemed to be analogous to the focus of our ultimate inquiry . . . in this way we distinguish our investigations from those which observe the natural event directly" (p. 106). Briefly, the limitations of the analogue method are (according to Maher 1966) the possible difficulty of ensuring that the analogue (either subject, situation, or behavior) shares the essential characteristics of the natural event and, second, the ultimate necessity of confirming hypotheses in the natural environment. Farber (1968) expressed the former limitation as follows: ". . . before one generalizes from observations of behavior in the laboratory to real-life situations, one had better consider very carefully the differences between the laboratory conditions and those in real life" (p. 161). Brunswik (1947) coined the term *ecological validity*[a] to refer to an extremely important criterion of meaningful experimentation: appropriate generalization from the laboratory to nonexperimental situations.

In our discussion of the psychology of illness, we saw how a person becoming ill and ultimately assuming the sick-role can undergo a number of important psychological changes. Experimental analogues of the placebo effect are minimal in ecological validity when they do not use patients as subjects, for healthy people usually do not undergo any form of therapy—that is, they do not take two aspirins in the absence of symptoms or see a therapist in the absence of psychological distress. There are important differences in subjects, situations, *and* behaviors between laboratory studies of the placebo effect and studies of the placebo effect in its natural setting, and these differences are important enough to warrant being acknowledged, rather than being denied or even simply being ignored.

Garfinkel (1967) has pointed out that the very nature of the psychological experiment means that it is episodic. As a consequence, it is not regarded by those concerned as being part of their everyday life experience but rather quite isolated from it. Orne (1970), discussing Garfinkel's point, states:

---

[a]This term is the one we shall use henceforth, and I am indebted to Professor Martin Orne for bringing it to my attention.

It is implicitly understood that at the conclusion of the experiment the episode will be concluded and the individual will be basically unchanged. Fears expressed, actions undertaken, emotions felt in the context of an experiment are experienced as specific to that situation and intended not to carry over beyond it. . . . Yet we hope to use our observations obtained in episodic situations to draw meaningful inferences about enduring motives of individuals as they manifest themselves in non-episodic contexts [pp. 188-189].

Fears expressed, actions undertaken, and emotions felt by patients who are hoping to get well and who may be in situations of considerable stress are simply not the same as those of healthy college sophomores who spend three hours in a laboratory, swallow two pink pills, perform a number of psychomotor tasks, and get paid five dollars and have a few points added to their introductory psychology course final examination score for their trouble. Even then, the placebo effect might be influenced by a host of factors that must be considered, but are not taken care of in the experimental design, for Orne has shown that when the object of study is an active, sentient human being, his or her awareness of the process of study may interact with the parameters under study. There are many ways in which artifact can creep into an experiment and introduce a number of factors that not only make it somewhat less "kosher" than it might be, but also make the consideration of the experiment's ecological validity even more difficult. The problem of demand characteristics, which will be discussed in more detail in a later chapter, is of considerable importance here; the demand characteristics of experiments using nonpatient subjects may be quite different from those involved when the subject is a patient who hopes that taking the medication or submitting to the therapeutic procedure of whatever nature will relieve his or her distress.

This discussion does not mean that we should abandon experimentation completely, for that might mean that our studies will become uncontrolled shambles and even veritable orgies of every thing the word "unscientific" implies. What it does mean is that we should think of how we can best approach maximum ecological validity. Nothing prevents us from conducting a greater number of experiments in the subjects' habitat and fewer in the nonpatient laboratory where precision under the circumstances outlined above is often illusory. Nothing prevents us from introducing into patient situations a number of manipulations of independent variables and a number of measures in such a way that by being as unobtrusive as possible we are not making ourselves into unwarranted and perhaps suspect disturbers of the situations in which patients find themselves. The greater the extent to which the dependent variables under study are nonspecific, the more we have to recognize how exquisite are the phenomena with which we are dealing and how more naturalistic experimentation will allow us to maximize ecological validity and hence the veridicality of our data. In the next chapter we shall continue our search for the parameters of the placebo effect with a consideration of studies using placebos in situations where ecological validity *is* maximal—that is, clinical studies in which the subjects of inquiry are patients.

5

Studies of Placebo Effects in Clinical Situations

Studies conducted on the placebo effect in clinical situations can obviously not be criticized on the basis of a lack of ecological validity, since therapeutic drugs are not routinely administered in situations in which there is no presenting complaint of a medical, surgical, or psychological nature. In this chapter, we shall look at a number of studies, most of which have been designed not to test hypotheses but rather to assess the effects of placebo treatment in one condition or another. These conditions include placebo effects in medical and surgical patients and placebo effects in a variety of psychiatric situations. There is an appreciable difference between the volume of work published in these two areas, with an overwhelming preponderance of literature concentrating on psychiatric, rather than medical or surgical, situations. An obvious reason for this difference is that in medical and surgical situations we are dealing with factors whose etiology is usually specific enough to warrant intervention by a specific agent; thus in medicine, an antibiotic will destroy microbial infection and in surgery a laryngectomy will remove a cancerous larynx. These are specific effects: A placebo will neither destroy *E. coli* nor eliminate the cancer. Placebos may, however, be effective in the relief of a number of symptoms such as the pain and the psychological distress that, as we have seen in the previous two chapters, will probably accompany these conditions. In psychiatric situations we are not dealing with such specific examples of the medical model; hence the role played by nonspecific effects is much greater.

Placebo Effects in Medicine and Surgery

That placebos may induce subtle physiological changes that parallel the subjective experiences described by the subject was demonstrated, in a study where n equalled 1, by Wolf and Wolff, as long ago as 1943. Their patient's stomach, which was permanently exposed to view following an accident, was observed after he ingested various drugs. Acid secretion and the appearance of the organ were studied, and the investigators found that even after the `administration of "three large imposing-looking red capsules" (Claridge 1972, p. 29), the patient experienced abdominal discomfort and the folds of his stomach became red and inflamed. A similar reaction, as well as a marked increase in stomach acid secretion, was caused by an injection of distilled water.

Braunstein and Moscone (1964) administered placebos to ninety-six patients on surgical and clinical wards in a hospital for three days and reported the following (as quoted from the abstract of their article that originally appeared in Spanish): "Half the patients were then asked questions about the effects suggesting depressive effects, and the other half questions suggesting excitatory effects. Results indicated: suggestion can be produced just by the questions asked, even under double-blind conditions; this occurs more readily for believing in the 'depressive' quality of the drug; autosuggestion in the drug administrator has a definite influence on the results; and the autosuggestion has no influence if only the subject's report is taken and no questions are asked." Again, the important effects that types of questions asked, checklist items, and so forth can have on reported results must be stressed (cf. the studies of Brodeur 1965 and Gowdey et al. 1967).

Batterman and Lower (1968) administered analgesic placebo therapy to 173 patients suffering from various musculoskeletal complaints. Placebos were administered in an "open trial"—that is, the study was not double-blind. In patients suffering from osteoarthritis, placebo responsiveness was high, and its extent was correlated with the amount of previous (principally analgesic) therapy. The proportion of patients with no previous therapy who responded to the placebo was 34.9 percent, that of those for whom previous therapy had been ineffective was 29.1 percent, while 77.9 percent of those for whom therapy in a previous situation had been effective in its first week, 40 percent of those for whom previous therapy had been effective in its second week, and 35 percent of those for whom previous therapy had been effective in its third week responded to placebo. For patients suffering from rheumatoid arthritis, the results were somewhat different: Only 15.7 percent of those who had had no previous therapy responded to the analgesic placebo, none at all whose previous therapy was ineffective responded, while 54.5 percent of those for whom previous therapy had been effective in its first week, 36.3 percent of those for whom previous therapy had been effective in its second week, and 26.1 percent of those for whom previous therapy had been effective in its third week responded to the analgesic placebo. Clearly, responsiveness to placebo therapy was related to effectiveness of previous therapy. Responsiveness to placebo therapy was also related to type of diagnosis and race: Caucasian patients retained responsiveness for three weeks if osteoarthritis was the diagnosis, while black patients were more likely to retain placebo responsiveness for both osteo- and rheumatoid-arthritic conditions.

In their book, *Placebos et effet placebo en médecine,* Kissel and Barrucand (1964) present a number of instances in which placebos were used with medical patients whose complaints included among others cardiovascular, pulmonary, endocrine, and rheumatic diseases, as well as a number of surgical cases including, for example, mock ligation of the internal mammary artery. These authors cited a table (adapted from Haas, Fink, and Härtfelder 1959) summarizing placebo effectiveness (positive placebo effect) in different symptoms.

Some of these data for the literature up to 1959 are: a mean of 28.2 percent for twenty-five studies of analgesia, 32.3 percent for five studies of migraine, 58 percent in a study of seasickness, 41 percent for two studies of cough relief, 49 percent for eight studies of rheumatism, and 24 percent for four studies of dysmenorrhea and menopausal complaints.

The literature on the nonpsychiatric uses of placebos is not as voluminous as the literature on psychiatric uses. The efficacy of placebos in medicine and surgery is impressive, however, and reinforces the remark made by Harrison quoted earlier in this book that "the only patient who can present a malady due solely to structural disease is an unconscious patient" (Harrison 1963, p. 4).

FURTHER EXPLANATION NEEDED

The Placebo Effect in Psychiatry

The ever-increasing use of drugs in the treatment of a host of psychiatric conditions, and the clinical efficacy of a large percentage of such drugs, has led to a situation in which many are routinely administered as a standard part of psychiatric practice. One should not, however, get completely carried away by their success, for as Fisher (1970a) has remarked, unfortunately when a standard psychotropic drug is standardly prescribed, very reliable results cannot be predicted. One might hope that the patients would respond in a standard, predictable way, whereas in fact they will behave with great variability. "If one compares . . . the predictability of various psychotropic agents with, for example, the specificity of quinidine in the treatment of cardiac arrhythmias, the efficacy of propylthiouracil for thyrotoxicosis, or even the use of tetracyclines for bacterial infections, it becomes clear that the therapeutic outcome following the administration of psychiatric drugs seems to depend upon many more factors than are usually encountered in other areas of clinical medicine" (Fisher 1970a, pp. 17-18). These comments point very strongly to the operation of a number of nonspecific factors even in the administration of active drugs, and thus the appearance of a greater number of reports on the use of placebos in psychiatry than on their use in any other areas of medicine is not surprising. In this section we shall examine the use of placebos in the treatment of a variety of psychiatric conditions including schizophrenia, depression, anxiety, and alcoholism.

Placebo Effects in Schizophrenic Patients

An examination of the literature on placebo effects in schizophrenic patients reveals a number of different opinions and different results concerning the appropriateness and efficacy, respectively, of such treatment. One of the difficulties encountered here might be the lack of specificity with which the word "schizophrenia" is used. The second edition of the *Diagnostic and Statistical Manual (DSM-II)* of the American Psychiatric Association (1968) lists thirteen types, including a "wastebasket" category. This sort of breakdown is seldom given in the literature to be reviewed here, and even though the fact is recognized that diagnostic difficulties in schizophrenia are appreciable, nonetheless we seldom find that any attempts at diagnoses finer than the label "schizophrenia" are made in the placebo studies.

A striking dependence on a placebo was demonstrated by Vinar (1969) in a forty-four-year-old periodically catatonic schizophrenic woman. Dramatic relief from headaches, insomnia, and anxiety was obtained by using a placebo (first pink and then blue pills twice daily) that was presented as a "new major tranquilizer" after several major tranquilizers (chlorpromazine, thioridazine, prochlorperazine) had proved to be ineffective. Without medical advice, the patient doubled the dose and then increased it even further until she was taking as many as nine tablets daily. Vinar always permitted an increase in the doze of placebo and only warned the patient that the higher the dose, the more danger there was of troublesome effects, but the patient always assured him that there were none. When the dose reached twelve tablets per day, the patient complained of anxiety and insomnia and an attempt was made to reduce the dose. A month later, the patient complained of sweating and inability to think and work for two days and confessed that she had been taking twenty-five tablets per day for several days and thus had had no tablets left for these last two days. After thoroughly discussing her life situation with her and satisfactorily intervening in the patient's employment situation to reduce her anxiety there, Vinar asked her to cut down her dosage to twelve tablets per day and two months later, to three tablets per day. Finally, an effective maintenance dosage of two tablets a day was reached. The patient displayed four of the five normal traits of drug dependence described by Staehelin (1960): a tendency to increase the dose, an inability to stop taking the tablets without psychiatric help, an almost compulsive desire to take the tablets, and withdrawal or abstinence syndrome on sudden deprivation of the "medication."

The study of Goldman, Witton, and Scherer (1965) mentioned previously in the discussion of the physical aspects of the placebo used as subjects thirty-two chronic schizophrenic males on two separate wards. These patients served simultaneously to test two hypotheses: first, that more reactions would be produced by a "drug" (placebo) given parenterally than one administered orally and, second, that a "drug" (placebo) said to activate behavior would have less effect than one said to deactivate behavior. The first hypothesis was not supported, but subjects were found to be suggestible to "treatments" designed to decrease rather than increase their ward activity, thereby implying, according to the investigators, that actual tranquilizers may have more of a placebo effect than actual antidepressants.

Bishop and Gallant (1966) found that in severely chronic patients, placebo responses and effects that enhanced medication were slight and transient, with no apparent relationship between the response to active compounds and that to placebo. Patients tended to respond to a second course of placebo with a worsening of clinical condition, thereby suggesting a limited nocebo effect with an inert agent. The ineffectiveness of placebo treatment in male schizophrenic patients was demonstrated in another study carried out by Hekimian and Friedhoff (1967). Thirty male schizophrenics were treated with placebo, chlorpromazine, or chlordiazepoxide. The placebo effect was minimal, while chlorpromazine was the most effective treatment. Chlordiazepoxide was effective enough for four out of ten patients to be discharged, while all treated with chlorpromazine, and none treated with placebos, were dischargeable.

A number of studies on the effectiveness of placebos in outpatients visiting a drug clinic were carried out by Lowinger and Dobie (1969). The studies were performed in the larger context of drug evaluations (each with a placebo control) and had a percentage of schizophrenic subjects ranging from 30 percent to 50 percent (no specification of schizophrenic type was given by the authors), with the remainder being divided between personality disorders and psychoneurosis, depending on the particular study. Placebo response rates ranged from 24 percent to 76 percent in the four studies, but unfortunately no breakdown of the placebo responsivity for each category was given. A study published in 1960 by Hankoff, Freedman, and Engelhardt gave results of schizophrenic patients treated with placebos in an outpatient setting. No differentiation of diagnosis of the 103 patients was given by the investigators, other than the label "schizophrenia." A placebo response was seen in forty-two patients, no response in forty-one, and a nocebo response in twenty. Dropout or hospitalization, viewed as treatment "failure," correlated with the absence of a placebo response: 86.8 percent of the patients failing to show a placebo response were considered treatment failures, and 54.7 percent of those showing a placebo response were also characterized in this way.

A paper presented at the Fourth World Congress of Psychiatry in Madrid, 1966, by Cole, Bonato, and Goldberg (1968) reported on two large collaborative studies developed by the psychopharmacology program of NIMH to evaluate phenothiazines in newly hospitalized schizophrenic patients. The first study involved 344 patients who had been randomly assigned to chlorpromazine, thioridazine, fluphenazine, and placebo for a six-week treatment period, with a one-year followup period after patients' release from the hospital. In the second study, patients were randomly assigned chlorpromazine, fluphenazine, and acetophenazine, and their progress was followed in or out of hospital for twenty-six weeks. Two major patient characteristics, race and sex, showed significant relationships to drug versus placebo response: Female acute schizophrenics improved more on drug treatment and less on placebo than male schizophrenics, and black schizophrenics not only did as well on drugs as white patients but also had a better response rate on placebo. According to the authors, if one equates nonspecific factors with improvement during treatment on placebos, the data indicate that "paranoid and related symptoms, which might be considered similar to Bleuler's secondary symptoms of schizophrenia, show moderate improvement on placebo but show significantly more improvement on phenothiazine treatment. Symptoms such as indifference to environment or hebephrenic giggling and grimacing which may be similar to Bleuler's primary symptoms, show essentially no change on placebo but significant improvement on phenothiazines" (Cole et al. 1968 pp. 117-18). The phrase "nonspecific factors" refers, of course, not only to placebos but also to other factors such as ward milieu. Paranoid symptoms in the placebo group were also found to be significantly affected by ward characteristics, and symptoms related to withdrawal were not.

Regarding rehospitalization of patients, this study found that assignment to the placebo during the six-week inhospital period decreased the likelihood of rehospitalization, as did phenothiazines and/or psychotherapy after discharge. The investigators examined possible causes (including differential discharge from the hospital and a number of other possible artifacts) for the effect of placebo treatment in decreasing rehospitalization, and only two significant differences between drug- and placebo-treated patients were revealed: Placebo patients were hospitalized for an average of six weeks longer than patients who had received an active drug treatment, and patients who received placebo or chlorpromazine were more likely to have fathers who were mentally ill than were patients receiving fluphenazine or thioridazine. Since, however, father's illness increased the likelihood of rehospitalization, these patients would have been more, rather than less, likely to have been rehospitalized. The authors speculated that the extended hospitalization that the placebo patients experienced might have been due to the fact that since they improved less during the six-week double-blind study than the drug patients, they were thought by the staff to be receiving placebos (which thus broke the double-blind), and consequently, the staff "responded to the 'deprived' patient[s] with some special quality in care, treatment or concern" (Cole et al. 1968, p. 124). An important note here is that although this study was conducted at nine collaborating hospitals, the particular hospital at which the patient was treated was found to have absolutely no relationship with drug-placebo differences.

As is apparent from these findings, the effectiveness of placebos in the treatment of schizophrenia is, for a number of reasons, widely variable. The label "schizophrenia" has been somewhat loosely applied in most of the studies mentioned above, so that the seriousness and type of the disorder may have varied widely in the patients treated in each study. The effectiveness of placebos was greater in outpatients (Vinar 1969; Lowinger and Dobie 1969; Hankoff et al. 1960) and low (Bishop and Gallant 1966) to virtually nonexistent (Hekimian and Friedhoff 1967) in chronic, hospitalized patients. Possibly the outpatients were not only less seriously disturbed, but were also more susceptible to nonspecific effects related to factors in their lives over which little control could be exercised by the investigators and which could have affected the dependent variables.

Caffey, Hollister, Kaim, and Pokorny (1971) have said that "placebos or control substances . . . produce little mean improvement in groups of schizo-phrenic patients: some individuals improve slightly, but an equal amount become worse. The changes produced by antipsychotic drugs are different from and more specific than in those patients who improved when treated with placebo" (p. 432). Until we know a great deal more about schizophrenia (both its nature and its treatment), and in view of the grave ethical implications of placebo treatment in schizophrenia, such treatment should, at least as a matter of routine, be conducted only with the utmost caution.

Placebos in Affective Disorders: Depression

An important distinction should be made here between symptoms of depression that are part of a larger constellation of psychiatric symptoms and the psychiatric diagnosis of depression, either reactive or endogenous. "Of all the symptoms complained of by the mentally ill patient, depression is certainly the most common. A melancholic mood can, of course, accompany any mental (or physical) illness. As a psychiatric diagnosis, however, depression refers to the condition in which the change in mood forms the major part of the patient's psychological state" (Claridge 1972, p. 165). Despite the clinical and biological differences that, according to Akiskal and McKinney (1973) have been described for the various categories of depression, many symptoms (psychomotor and vegetative dysfunction, dysphoria, hopelessness, suicidal preoccupation) that constitute the syndrome of depression are common to the entire group of depressive disorders. Therefore, problems can arise when, as we shall see, admission to a study is based on symptoms rather than diagnosis.

Honigfeld (1968), in a paper on specific and nonspecific factors in the treatment of depressed states, presented at the Fourth World Congress of Psychiatry, Madrid, 1966, indicated that "well-controlled studies and a wealth of clinical data support the role of drug therapy and selective electroshock therapy in depressed patients. Furthermore, the superiority of the new chemical agents to earlier forms of somatic therapy, placebo therapy or no therapy has been amply demonstrated" (p. 80). Honigfeld pointed out that a particular problem faces the researcher or therapist who uses placebos in the treatment of psychiatrically diagnosed depression: Cyclic fluctuations and spontaneous remis-sions are part of the natural course of affective disorders, and unless a no-treatment condition is included in any research design, the so-called placebo effects might well be nothing more than natural fluctuations observed during placebo treatment that are not due to placebo administration.

Honigfeld also stressed the importance of clearly specifying the diagnostic composition of groups under study, since depressive disorders do vary in terms of prognosis and expected response to treatment. A number of types of affective disorders, whose common core phenomenon is depressive mood, were listed by Honigfeld (1968) whose discussion on classification and treatment of such disorders was based on the investigations by Klein and his associates (the reader is referred to the references at the end of Honigfeld's article for details of the sources of Klein's published works). The classification of affective disorders were as follows: retarded depressions, manic states, agitated depressions, reactive and neurotic depressive reactions, emotionally unstable character disorders, and phobic anxiety reactions. The very specific therapeutic effects of drug treatment in most affective disorders was mentioned. In most depressive disorders, when placebos are used we find a roughly normal distribution of therapeutic response. In retarded depressions, however, this therapeutic response distribution is more likely to be bimodal, so that we are possibly dealing with two subclassifications within this category: one group exhibiting no change and the other showing good response under placebo treatment. The latter group might also be composed of two subgroups: those in whom what is observed is the spontaneous course of the disorder (i.e., not a placebo effect) and those who are responding to the placebo. However, this finer subdivision cannot be made without having patients who are no-treatment controls.

With the above in mind, we can turn to a study by Malitz and Kanzler (1971). The aim of the study was to evaluate the antidepressant qualities of a number of antidepressant drugs and a placebo. The antidepressant drugs (diphenyldantoin, dextroamphetamine, amitriptyline-perphenazine, amitriptylene-diazepam, nortriptyline, AY-62014, and amitriptylene) had not previously been compared with each other or with a placebo in terms of relative effectiveness as antidepressants, although antidepressant effects had been claimed for them largely on the basis of studies omitting a placebo group. The subjects were 312 patients referred to a psychiatry medication clinic over a period of about four years; 203 patients completed the study. Admission to the study was on the basis of symptoms of depression. About 70 percent of the patients were considered to be acutely ill (symptoms present for less than two years), and the remainder were chronic. Treatment was double-blind, and patients were randomly assigned to one of thirteen psychiatrists. Treatment consisted of one week of placebo and four weeks of active substance for seven of the eight treatment groups; the eighth group received placebo throughout the five weeks. Patients were required to visit the physician at the end of each week of treatment. Formal evaluations of their condition were made at the first (pretreatment) and sixth (posttreatment) visits. The twelve variables considered relevant in assessing improvement were: global scales of degree of mental illness, anxiety, and depression; the Brief Psychiatric Rating Scale (PBRS) subscales of somatic concern, anxiety, guilt, tension, depressive mood, and motor retardation; and the MMPI, Scale 2 (D) and the Taylor Manifest Anxiety subscales. Out of the eighty-four comparisons made between placebo and active treatment (twelve relevant variables, seven comparisons on each) only four showed significant positive results in which the drug was superior to the placebo, and eleven showed significant negative results. The effectiveness of the placebos in the relief of target symptoms was striking.

Unfortunately, the investigators assessed the effects of the various treatments only in relation to the target symptoms and not to the psychiatric diagnostic categories into which the patients were divided. We therefore have no information about the effectiveness of any treatment in this study in relation, for example, to the types of depression that were mentioned by Honigfeld (1968). It is true, as Malitz and Kanzler (1971) stated, that "unless [a placebo group is included in drug evaluation studies] many drugs will continue to receive the credit for producing improvement that really reflects spontaneous remission, the natural course of the disorder, or perhaps, the psychotherapeutic skill of the treating physician" (p. 1610). But since these factors were not controlled or even documented by them, we cannot, from their study, draw any conclusions about the effectiveness of placebos in the treatment of depression. In addition, as Wainwright wrote in the discussion postscripted at the end of the Malitz and Kanzler article, "validation is not assured statistically when it is based only on target symptoms" and at least some attempt at classification would be desirable in order to increase the value of a study such as this one.

Clearly, then, a study that includes a no-treatment condition in order to control for the confounding factors that Honigfeld mentioned and also makes *some* attempt at using diagnostic groups is necessary before we can say anything further about how effective placebos are in the treatment of depression. We should give Malitz and Kanzler due credit, however, for they did recognize the former problem, and their study was not, in any case, designed to show that placebos do work. Vinar (1968), in a discussion at the Fourth World Congress of Psychiatry, Madrid, 1966, stated that in his hospital every patient was routinely administered placebos under double-blind conditions for at least a week after admission and that eighteen of two hundred depressed patients improved after they were treated unsuccessfully for long periods of time with antidepressant drugs. According to Vinar (1968):

These patients recovered soon after the antidepressant medication was replaced by a placebo. While the possibility of spontaneous remission cannot fully be discounted, we have, however, the clinical impression that antidepressant drugs, continuously administered for long periods of time for some patients, may retard the onset of spontaneous remissions. We believe that, in some patients at least, the long-term administration of . . . antidepressant drugs should suddenly be interrupted by a placebo interval [p. 132].

Even this limited usefulness of placebos indicates the need that exists for a great deal of further research on their effects in the treatment of psychoses and affective disorders.

Placebo Effects in the Treatment of Anxiety

Excessive anxiety may disrupt a person's usual coping mechanisms in such a way that he or she becomes tense, phobic, inhibited by fear, and socially withdrawn. When anxiety is sufficiently high to interfere with adaptive functioning, antianxiety agents are useful for what Shader (1970) called "unlock [ing] frozen ego resources" (p. 71). The minor tranquilizers are probably the most widely prescribed of all psychoactive agents. Many studies using placebos in the place of antianxiety agents have shown the remarkable effectiveness of the former. For example, twenty-nine anxious patients were studied by Black (1966). Fourteen of these received placebos, and fifteen received sodium amylobarbitone. Progress, judged by Hamilton's Anxiety State Rating Scale, was parallel for both groups; hence no specific drug effect was demonstrated. Age and sex did not relate to improvement, but patients ill for less than a year improved most.

The factors that account for the great effectiveness of placebos as anxiolytics are complex. The case is not simply one of administering placebos and then having the patient's anxiety reduced. The effectiveness of placebos is related to many factors, such as the instructions given to the patient, who the treating physician is, and how the physician behaves. These factors will all be discussed later in this book in the sections on the prognostic uses of placebos, the personality of the placebo reactor, and situational analyses of the placebo effect. In order to avoid repetition and, more importantly, to illustrate the complexity of the factors leading to the obtained effect, the studies dealing with these issues are not included here and the interested reader is urged to consult the sections mentioned above.

Placebo Effects in the Treatment of Alcoholism

"The prevention and treatment of alcoholism represents a public health problem for psychiatry which exceeds in numbers and consequences the problems related to all of the other drugs combined" (Meyer 1970, p. 258). Whether patients are acute or chronic alcoholics, skid-row bums, or aristocrats, the consequences of their drinking, both to themselves and in relation to the larger social sequelae (in the family, at work, in an automobile on the road), can be so grave that extensive research into their management, treatment, and cure is essential. Treatment of alcoholism per se, without examining the patient's anxieties, depressions, and the reasons why he or she drinks is not, as Meyer (1970) points out, very successful: "Alcoholic behavior is merely the end stage of a life history. Moreover, one-shot aversive techniques constitute 'punishment,' and learning theorists point out that behavior is not extinguished by punishment" (p. 260). The multiplicity of treatments available suggests that no one treatment is really effective, but in view of the complexity of syndromes present in any single patient or group of patients (with manifold pharmacological, sociological, and psychological interactions), the failure of simplistic "cookbook" or "recipe" approaches is not surprising. How effective are placebos in the treatment of alcoholism, and is their use justified?

An experiment by Smart and Bateman (1967) was mentioned by Barber (1970). The investigators randomly assigned thirty alcoholic patients at a Toronto clinic to one of three treatments: the standard treatment used for alcoholics at the clinic; the standard treatment plus one session in which the patient received a very high (800 micrograms) dose of LSD-25; and the standard treatment plus one session in which the patient received an active placebo. About 80 percent of the patients showed a reduction of alcohol intake after each of the three treatments: They did not differ significantly in abstinence or amount of drinking at a six-month and also a two-year posttreatment evaluation. "The LSD treatment reduced the amount of drinking in this investigation to the same degree as in earlier investigations, but the reduction was no greater than that produced by ephedrine or by the standard treatment alone" (Barber 1970, p. 58). The same results were obtained for placebo treatment as for the other two treatments, and in view of the fact that the placebo was only given once, whether the placebo treatment per se contributed anything at all to treatment outcome is doubtful. Great care must be exercised in adducing to the placebo treatment more effectiveness than it warrants.

Two interesting studies on the treatment of alcoholism with placebos have been reported in the Soviet literature. Yalovoy (1969) used a substitute for the alcohol-Antabuse test in treating alcoholism with calcium glycerophosphate placebos. Antabuse is a substance that when taken prior to ingestion of alcohol, produces a reaction that typically includes flushing, redness of the eyes, slight hypertension, severe tachycardia, a sense of apprehension, a pounding headache, and rapid breathing. Antabuse produces an extremely aversive reaction syndrome to alcohol. Yalovoy studied two groups: one receiving Antabuse and one receiving placebo. Satisfactory results (abstinence from alcohol for at least four to six months after treatment) were obtained; these results were identical for both groups, despite the fact that there was a predominance of the more seriously ill among those receiving the placebo.

The other Soviet study was reported by Zvonikov (1969) who presented a modification of the technique for conditional reflex therapy of alcoholism based on apomorphine (a prompt and effective emetic) and suggestion.[a] Patients were called one by one into the treatment room, and an apomorphine solution (0.3 gm) of effective strength was administered in the form of an injection, while others received injections of 0.1 gm apomorphine (ineffectively small), or placebo (Vitamin B_1). The patients were, of course, unaware of these treatment

[a]The procedure used in this study, which appeared in *Soviet Neurology and Psychiatry*, 3 (1969):66-71, was not very cogently presented, and I have written to Zvonikov for further details of his work, but have not at the time of this writing received a reply.

differences. Then the doctor called to his table each of the patients who had received the 0.3 gm dose of apomorphine and gave each a glass of water to drink and a small piece of cotton moistened with vodka to smell. The doctor immediately began making appropriate suggestions about the appearance of autonomic reactions and nausea. When the autonomic reactions appeared, small doses of vodka were offered to the patient. Suggestion was continued, and an intensification of nausea and an onset of vomiting occurred. Nausea and vomiting continued in a considerable number of patients who had not been called to the doctor's table, even though they received placebos or ineffectively small doses of apomorphine. According to Zvonikov, the experiment showed that conditioned, emotionally negative and vomiting reactions to alcohol could be developed in a short period of time by using a placebo or very small doses of apomorphine (which was also, in effect, a placebo). In addition, remission was found to be maintained in 48.7 percent of the patients for more than two years.

A study carried out by Strassman, Adams, and Pearson (1970) on the effectiveness of metronidazole and placebo for the treatment of the so-called social drinker (who drinks too much on social occasions and for whom the rather insidious process of becoming an alcoholic might already have begun) revealed the ineffectiveness of placebos in curbing drinking. Surprisingly enough, however, none of the subjects taking the active drug reported psychological subjective side effects, while 44 percent of those receiving placebo did. These side effects were depression, "loggy feeling," "feel bad," and nervousness. The investigators did not comment on the nocebo effects, and in view of the dearth of information they presented, doing so here is not possible either.

Some argument is possible here on the use of the word *nocebo* for placebos that produce aversive effects such as those seen in some of the studies discussed in this section. The substitutes for the active agents have been referred to as *placebos* since the effects, even though aversive, were directly concerned with the target symptoms under consideration. In order to avoid as much confusion as possible, I prefer reserving the term *nocebo* for side or incidental effects when these are noxious, and not for the expected effects even when these are noxious.

The findings of these studies indicate that in situations in which the treatment of choice for alcoholism is based on the aversive conditioning paradigm, placebos can be effective substitutes for active pharmacological agents. Where the treatment for alcoholism does not include an additional pharmacological agent, placebos do not add anything to the effectiveness of that treatment, nor are they apparently effective in the treatment of prealcoholism drinking behavior. Further research in this area is clearly necessary before anything that even approaches a recommendation for a standard treatment for particular cases can be made, but we can say that in cases where active pharmacological agents are contraindicated at least an attempt at placebo treatment seems justified.

Prognostic Uses of Placebos

Several authors have carried out investigations based on the general hypothesis that some persons will show a general, favorable tendency to respond positively to treatment (in particular, psychiatric treatment) and that such persons can be identified on the basis of their responses to placebos, which are a symbol of the process of treatment rather than a physical, active pharmacological treatment per se.

A frequently cited experiment by Hankoff, Freedman, and Engelhardt (1958) was one of the first to relate placebo reactivity to the effectiveness of subsequent treatment. Thirty-three schizophrenic patients were treated for three months with placebos and later on standard medication. Fifteen of the patients were placebo reactors, and eighteen were not. Among the patients, seven who were placebo-resistant had to be rehospitalized almost immediately. Nine of the fifteen who had to be rehospitalized one to nine months after treatment were placebo reactors. Eleven showed good results for one and a half to two years after treatment; of these, nine were placebo reactors. This study concluded that the probability of a favorable placebo response seems like a prognostic sign of future success in the maintenance of an ambulatory state. "Hankoff [et al.] confirmed their results in 1960. [They] treated 103 patients, of whom 42 were placebo reactors, and noted that only 13.1 percent of the patients who did not react to placebos reacted to the standard treatment, and 86.9 percent of these subjects experienced treatment failure" (Kissel and Barrucand 1964, p. 160, my translation). This second study by Hankoff et al. (1960) was mentioned earlier in this chapter in the section on the use of placebos in treating schizophrenia and as might be noticed, Kissel and Barrucand, in reporting it, have made slight but not significant, alterations in the percentages they cited.

Glick (1967) attempted to examine the relationship between the placebo response and clinical outcome on an active drug (perphenazine). Twenty psychiatric patients with varied diagnoses were treated for two weeks with placebo, followed by four weeks with perphenazine. The first hypothesis, that subjects developing side effects on the placebo would not do as well on the active medication as those not developing side effects, was confirmed. The second hypothesis, that patients improving clinically on placebo would do better on active drug than those not improving, was not confirmed. No significant relationship between the presence and absence of side effects while on placebos and active drugs was found.

Shapiro, Wilensky, and Struening (1968) conducted an experiment using a "placebo test"—essentially a measurement of acute placebo reactivity—on twenty-seven patients of varied diagnoses in a psychiatry outpatient clinic. Subjects were given a tablet and asked to record changes at least every fifteen minutes for one hour. Rating of the placebo test was as follows: The responses of a positive reactor for the first fifteen minutes included such statements as "headache decreasing," "nervousness gone," and "feeling better"; those for a negative reactor included "feel like vomiting now" and "feel nauseous and my eyesight is blurred"; while neutral reactors said things such as "no effect yet" and "no effect." Each statement was classified as positive, negative, or neutral by two independent judges (correlations ranged from +.90 to +.98), and each subject was classified as positive, negative, or neutral according to the greatest number of positive, negative, or neutral statements on the placebo test. Reaction to the placebo test was 26 percent positive, 26 percent neutral, and 48 percent negative. Third-year residents then treated patients in the psychopharmacology clinic. Although the main emphasis was on drug treatment, other appropriate therapies were used concurrently. Formal followup evaluations were scheduled at three, six, and twelve months, as well as two years later. The correlation coefficient was +.87 for ratings of improvement made on a seven-point scale at three months by two independent judges, and ratings were derived from conference reports and progress notes.

The hypothesis that positive, negative, and neutral placebo reactions would correlate with improved, worse, and unimproved clinical courses, respectively, was partially supported. Positive placebo reactors improved rapidly and maintained their improvement, neutral reactors improved less but maintained achieved improvement, and negative placebo reactors improved more slowly but reached the level of improvement of the neutral reactors at six months. To test whether variables other than the placebo test were related to improvement, correlation coefficients were computed for improvement and thirty-five other variables. "Negative correlations were obtained between improvement and duration of current illness, previous treatment, previous episodes of mental illness, and high scores on the Discomfort Symptom Scales. Further analysis indicated that less of the variance was explained by these variables than by the placebo test. Again, there is support for the conclusion that the placebo effect is a multi-determined, rather than a simple unidetermined phenomenon" (Shapiro et al. 1968, p. 128).

Rickels, Lipman, and Raab (1966) examined data collected in several of the studies they conducted. In a series of crossover studies, data on patients who received placebos after being on drug treatment during the first study phase were collected. The patient's presenting symptoms were not mentioned by the authors, but in view of the active drugs prescribed, presumably (from Appleton 1971), a major symptom was anxiety (see Appleton 1971 for an excellently organized and tabulated usage guide for psychoactive drugs). In the first phase, drugs were divided into therapeutically "active" drugs (meprobamate, chlordiazepoxide) that differ significantly from placebo and clinically "inactive" drugs (hydroxyzine, amphenidone, phenobarbital sodium). On subsequent placebo treatment, a 66 percent improvement rate was noted in patients (n = 29) who had initially received the "active" medication. "In other words, when offering a patient the possibility for a direct comparison between drugs, he frequently differentiates between active agent and placebo, and the more effective clinically the first agent, the worse is the subsequent placebo response" (Rickels, Lipman, and Raab, 1966, p. 549). In another study, the authors treated anxious neurotic medical clinic patients double-blind on either chlordiazepoxide (40 mg per dose) or placebo in identical capsules for four weeks, after which half the patients received Librium capsules in commercial Librium bottles for two weeks (Librium is a trade name for chlordiazepoxide) and the other half received identical placebos in the same fashion. Study physicians and the study nurse were all told that the bottles contained 10 mg Librium capsules and that the investigators wished to find out how patients would respond to "regular Librium" after having participated in the double-blind study for four weeks. Patients and physicians independently rated symptom reduction. The results showed that when dividing patients (irrespective of treatment) into improved and unimproved groups, the largest subsequent Librium-placebo difference in the clinical responses was found in patients who had responded positively to any of the prior medications. "Apparently, improved patients perceived the subsequent placebo as inactive and consequently did poorer than patients who were initially unimproved. This is also evident in the fact that of 14 dosage deviations occuring during this study phase, 11 occurred on placebo; and nine of these patients did not improve" (Rickels 1966, p. 549). The study also found that the degree of improvement observed on prior medication primarily affected subsequent placebo response and not drug response: Placebo patients of the initially improved group did significantly poorer than placebo patients of the initially unimproved group irrespective of prior medication.

Studying the effects of previous medication, Rickels, Lipman, and Raab, (1966) distinguished between "previous medication," which referred to all psychiatric drugs the patient had taken during the last several years, and "prior medication," which referred to medication the patient had received in the first treatment phase of the crossover studies. Patients were drawn from private psychiatric and private general practices and from clinics. The treatments were chlordiazepoxide, meprobamate, phenobarbital sodium, LA-1, a chlordiazepoxide analogue, and a placebo. The largest drug-placebo differences were observed in patients who had been previously treated with one or more of the drugs. While drug response was not influenced by previous medication, placebo response was: Patients with no or only one previous drug experience improved more on placebo than did patients with two or more previous drug experiences. Although the authors did not inquire whether a patient's previous drug experience had been of a positive or negative nature, they speculated that patients with several past drug experiences may have been better equipped to differentiate the active drugs from placebo. These investigators also found that patients who had been treated with several psychiatric drugs in the past were more chronically ill than those who had never been treated with psychiatric drugs. Acutely ill patients reported a comparatively high incidence of "no previous drug experience," while the more chronically ill patients reported a relatively high incidence of two or more previous drug experiences.

Dividing length of illness into categories of acute (up to six months) and subacute (seven to twelve months) plus chronic (over one year), the largest placebo-induced improvement was found in the acutely ill patients and the least placebo improvement in subacutely and chronically ill patients. Drug responses were, however, not significantly influenced by duration of illness. When using the patient's own global improvement ratings as criteria, no drug-placebo differences were found in the acutely ill patients. "In other words, chronicity affected drug-placebo differences in improvement rate by increasing the number of placebo-improved patients in the acute group, leading to insignificant drug-placebo differences in these patients, and by decreasing placebo-induced changes in the subacute and chronic patient group, producing significant drug-placebo differences" (Rickels, Lipman, and Raab, 1966, p. 552). Checking these findings with physicians' global improvement ratings, the researchers found that, in contrast to the patient's own ratings, the physicians' improvement ratings differentiated significantly between drug and placebo in the acutely ill patients; placebo patients were rated as doing more poorly. These data allow one to deduce that the placebo response is primarily present in the patient's own evaluation of change, particularly in the case of acutely ill patients. Patients overvalue their improvement, which therefore differs from the physician's more objective evaluation. In chronically ill patients, placebos have a less suggestive effect, so there tends to be more agreement between patients and physicians in regard to global improvement ratings. "This finding would lend support to the interpretation that the so-called 'positive placebo response' is often more a subjective than an objective or real one and therefore is more noticed by the patient in himself than by the more objective observer" (Rickels, Lipman, and Raab, 1966, p. 533).

The above experiment in particular and also the one by Shapiro et al. (1968) mentioned just before it allow us to be a little less cautious than Kissel and Barrucand were in 1964 when they wrote the following, with which we conclude this section on the prognostic uses of placebos: "Evidently it would be satisfying, based on the assumption that placebo-sensitivity is a characteristic of the normal subject, to also accept that it is, as a general rule, an indicator of a good prognosis. One cannot, in the meantime, justifiably deduce these conclusions from this principle, even if Hankoff's data seem valuable within the framework of his research. New experiments are now desirable and would allow there to be, ultimately, new clinical uses of the placebo. But, up to now, the use of placebos is essentially therapeutic" (p. 160, my translation).

Studies conducted to assess the response to treatment conditions usually involve the implementation of one or more treatment methods, which are then compared with each other or a no-treatment group on the basis of whichever posttreatment data are being considered. Provided that sufficient controls are included for other effects, researchers can conclude that their treatment, and not other effects, is a determinant of the observed therapeutic change. But in many cases, as we shall see in the following chapters, the influence of a number of other factors can be as important in the placebo effect as the actual treatment method. Most of these factors were not controlled in the studies we have examined up to this point, and after reading the following chapters, the reader will see that a persuasive argument for the almost mandatory control of many of these factors in *any* study on the placebo effect can be made. In any therapeutic situation, a patient and a therapist are both involved, and the interaction takes place with certain verbal behaviors and certain attitudes and perceptions in both parties. In the following chapters we shall examine how these are related to the placebo effect by starting, in the next chapter, with the personality of the patient undergoing treatment.

6 The Search for the Personality of the Placebo Reactor

The root of many of the nonspecific variables in treatment clearly lies in the person being treated, and as was emphasized in the introduction to this book, the role of the *person* must be considered in the treatment process. With the aid of the behavioral and social sciences, tomorrow's physicians, unlike so many of today's, must at least be able to see beyond a physical symptom to a person. A good starting point is the investigation of the personality of placebo reactors.

In this chapter we shall encounter a good share of the studies that have attempted such investigation by using psychometric instruments. Unfortunately, the number of studies designed specifically to this end has not been great. Many other studies, though, have included such psychometric assessment as an incidental part of the broader design; the results of the more noteworthy of these will be included here, too. We shall first consider some of the reasons for studying the personality of placebo reactors, and then we shall turn to an examination of the literature.

Reasons for Studying the Personality of Placebo Reactors

As has already been noted in this book, despite the large (and ever increasing) amount of literature published on the placebo effect in the last twenty years, we still have very little knowledge of its mechanism(s) of action. A large amount of the blame for this state of affairs can be attributed to the general lack of direction and the dearth of systematic research efforts in the area.

The first reason for studying the personality of placebo reactors is that since the placebo effect is a psychological phenomenon, subject variables and characteristics might throw a considerable amount of light on the adumbrated state of the theoretical explanations (alluded to in the preceding paragraph) that have been advanced for its modus operandi. This is particularly so in the case of theoretical explanations in which subject variables are an integral part of the explanatory factors and in which there is a correspondence between subject characteristics and a particular psychological mechanism (e.g., the experiments on body image, acquiescence, and perception of subjective changes following placebo ingestion, which we shall examine later in this chapter).

Second, such research might serve an important function in placebo therapy: The knowledge that certain personality types presenting certain symptoms might have a high probability of responding favorably to placebos would be extremely useful in cases where placebo administration is indicated as the treatment of preference rather than drugs. This reason is no less important than the first one given above. Just as an increasing number of drugs and medical treatments with a high degree of specificity and predictability have been developed, so, too, we might, by a series of investigations on placebo efficacy in a specified variety of complaints and in a variety of people, develop guidelines for the use of placebos—that is, guidelines that have a high degree of predictability of outcome. However, the fact should be reemphasized here that no matter how great the degree of specificity and predictability of active agents, the role of nonspecific factors—psychological ones—can never be excluded. In a like way, developing specificity and predictability for placebos will not necessarily make nonspecific factors unimportant even when placebos are used.

The third reason for studying the personality of the placebo reactor has been stated by Honigfeld (1964a): ". . . the evaluation of any form of therapy will be made more sensible by the elimination of subjects liable to respond to the non-specific components of the clinical trial situation" (p. 152). What Honigfeld was really talking about appears to be a triple-blind procedure, and for reasons pointed out earlier, triple-blind studies are of questionable value. Honigfeld's reason for studying placebo reactors' personality characteristics has therefore to be accepted with some reservation.

Claridge (1972) expressed the general nature of the research in this area rather well:

What is the popular notion of someone who is gullible enough to be taken in by a sugar pill and react to it as though given some potently active chemical? Probably that he (or more likely she!) is a weak minded hysteric, an unstable character over-concerned with bodily health. The truth is that extensive research has failed to identify any particular 'placebo type' who will respond to placebos consistently under all conditions. Instead of looking for such a global personality type, recent studies have tended to concentrate on rather more limited aspects of personality, seeing how they relate to the placebo response in narrowly defined situations. Research of this type has provided some evidence that certain personality characteristics may be found more commonly in placebo reactors than in non-reactors [pp.36-37].

Often, examining the data of subjects who do not perform in the hypothesized way in a particular experiment is a useful procedure. This "look-at-the-exceptions" rule of thumb can be applied here by looking not only at the placebo reactors, but also at the neutral or nonreactors and the negative reactors. Some researchers (e.g., Fisher and Olin 1956) reported that psychotic patients have more frequent negative reactions to placebos than do neurotics, but others have found only small or insignificant differences between the reactivity of psychotics and nonpsychotics (e.g., Kurland 1958). We can learn a lot about the mechanisms of placebo reactions by including data on both the characteristics of reactors *and* the other groups in our theoretical studies. We would be naive to assume that once we know who the placebo reactors are in a particular situation, the others can be defined by exclusion, so we will talk about nonreactors and negative reactors only when such subjects have been included in the data presentation, and we shall not make assumptions about them when we have no data with which to work. We will notice that the nonreactors and negative reactors have only infrequently been investigated in the studies we shall review.

We have already encountered Fisher's (1970) caution that "it is one thing to demonstrate that non-specific factors may influence drug response [but] it is a very different thing to conclude that the mechanism for the observed relationship must be equally non-specific in nature" (p. 19). Learning more about people who react to placebos in different ways can allow us to learn more about many of the nonspecific factors involved. Since, in truth, the human beings involved play an essential part in the placebo effect, we need not (unless we wish to be obtuse) look for further reasons for taking a look at their psychological natures by using standard (and some not-so-standard) psychological evaluation instruments.

The Research Literature

For purposes of clarity, the research literature will be considered under the following main headings:

The use of nonprojective personality instruments;

The use of projective personality instruments;

Suggestibility, acquiescence, hypnosis, and the placebo reactor;

Summary of the literature on the personality of the placebo reactor and some comments and conclusions.

Two important points should be noted prior to examining the studies themselves. The first is that many of the studies did not contain an explicit statement concerning the intention to assess the personality of placebo reactors; in many studies, this was quite incidental. The second point is that, ideally, the subjects in studies on the placebo effect should be patients rather than nonpatients or the ubiquitous college sophomore. The placebo effect is so complex that a true picture of either theoretical or practical value is more likely to be obtained in studies measuring the personalities of patients or of people self-administering nonprescription drugs. The psychology or psychopharmacology laboratory is a far cry from the patient-doctor-hospital milieu, the ecological validity of which is, for our purposes, so much higher than that of the former two settings.

The Use of Nonprojective Personality Instruments
in Assessing the Personality of Placebo Reactors

Studies in which the subjects were nonpatients. Muller (1965), in his report on a laboratory experiment using nonpatient subjects, attempted to justify studying such persons by stating that "several writers have suggested that more light might be shed on the placebo response if it could be studied in the laboratory rather than the clinic, so that factors involved could be systematically manipulated and their effects sorted out" (p. 58). Possible factors involved in the placebo response were systematically varied, and Muller's study used a nonstress experimental situation to determine (1) how consistent the individual reactions of normal subjects would be to repeated placebo administration, and (2) whether personality differences exist between consistent placebo reactors and nonreactors. The subjects were forty male, paid, volunteer college students, age twenty-one to twenty-three, each of whom had undergone a physical examination, completed the MMPI, and signed a release form. An initial "practice day" was followed by the subjects' reporting, at forty-eight-hour intervals, for six consecutive "drug" trials (inert placebo capsules). Each subject was pretested on a battery of psychophysiological tests, then given the "medication," following which the subject was kept occupied for forty-five minutes with various biographical questionnaires, interest inventories, and so forth. The subject was then posttested on the same battery of psychophysiological tests. Finally, each subject was interviewed and asked to complete a brief questionnaire concerning what subjective effects, if any, he had experienced following "medication."

Muller found, on the basis of subjects' scores on the measures of subjective placebo effects, that there was a bimodal distribution: Twelve subjects reported subjective effects on four to six placebo trials and were classified as reactors, while thirteen subjects reported zero to one subjective effect (the other end of the bimodal distribution) and were classified as nonreactors. The MMPI profiles of these two groups were compared. The composite profile (Hathaway code) of the reactor group was 93487, which is "indicative, in college males, of outgoing, verbally and socially skilled behavior, enthusiasm, and generally good adjustment, particularly in the area of social relations," and that of the nonreactors was 49837, which is "suggestive of an aggressive, belligerent personality, with marked antagonism for authority figures" (Muller 1965, p. 59). An essential characteristic of the Hathaway coding system is the use of primes and other signs to show the elevation of each scale in the profile. Since such signs were not included in Muller's article, we have little idea of the elevation (other than the means for Scales 4 and 9) and hence the significance of the scales in the composite profile. Significant differences were found between the mean scores of the two groups on both Scale 4 (reactors, $n = 23$, $Pd = 58.8$; non-reactors, $n = 17$, $Pd = 62.3$) and on Scale 9 (reactors, $n = 23$, $Ma = 64.3$; non-reactors, $n = 17$, $Ma = 59.3$). As will be noticed, twelve subjects were classified as "reactors" according to Muller's criterion, but $n = 23$ was presented in the data analysis. Likewise, thirteen subjects were classified as "nonreactors," but $n = 17$ was in the data analysis. Presumably, subjects falling in the middle of the bimodal distribution were included in the data analysis, although this was not stated by Muller. The statistical significance of the data presented must therefore be accepted with some doubt, especially because of the discrepancy for the reactor group ($n = 9$), and because fifteen apparently unclassified subjects were included in the data analysis.

Muller viewed his findings as supportive of the idea that a placebo administration involves the communication of expectations by an authority figure to a subordinate person and that the subordinate's personality and social adjustment are major determinants of the reception and acceptance of the communication. People with good social adjustment responded to the placebo, and people who exhibited a deviant social adjustment, particularly with reference to authority figures, showed no response. In my opinion, such an explanation is a far cry indeed from the medical milieu. Another criticism that can be made of all studies using volunteer subjects is that, as Rosenthal and Rosnow (1969) indicated, volunteer subjects often differ in significant ways from those who do not volunteer. Seriously biased estimates of various population parameters, and an interaction with experimental variables in such a way as to increase the probability of inferential Type I and Type II errors, can occur when using such subjects. Moreover, the type of subjects used (i.e., college sophomores) confirm McNemar's (1946 p. 33) lament that psychology is a science of sophomores, to which might again be added that the sophomores in this situation were not patients.

The basic procedural pattern of most experiments in this area is as follows: selection of subjects, who should ideally be patients; administration of the personality assessment device(s); pretest on one, or several, psychological laboratory tasks; pretest on subjective symptom checklist (which might conceivably be an important source of demand characteristics) or, preferably, a self-report of subjective symptoms; administration of placebo; posttest on subjective symptoms and note changes; selection of groups of placebo reactors, nonreactors, and nocebo reactors according to criteria determined on the basis of scores in the two posttests; examination of the personality test data of the groups selected. In some studies, additional data in the form of geographical, demographic, and other subject-specific information are obtained. Both pre- and posttests are essential if the scores of change after placebo are to be meaningful.

Unfortunately, the MMPI has hardly ever been used in experiments on placebos. Even a search through the literature on the use of the MMPI in studies of active drugs (e.g., all the references cited in Butcher 1969, pp. 350-51) revealed no data (because of the double-blind nature of some of the studies) on the personality attributes of the control subjects who in some cases received placebos. In one of the studies, by Haertzen and Hill (1959), MMPI data on the control subjects were presented, but whether or not they received placebos was not explicitly stated.

Joyce (1959) used the Bernreuter scale in his study and found that consistent placebo reactors (defined as those who showed a placebo reaction on two occasions) were less "self-confident" and "socially dominant," although they also tended to be more "social" and "extraverted." In a second phase of this investigation, Joyce used these findings on the Bernreuter scale to predict responses to placebos in a new group of subjects and was able to predict such responses at well beyond chance. All of Joyce's subjects were medical students, and not patients.

Other nonprojective devices, besides the MMPI and Bernreuter, have been used in investigations in this area. An overwhelming majority of them have been questionnaires and tests constructed by the investigators themselves, rather than widely used and well-validated psychological instruments. Sharp (1965) administered to eighty-eight subjects (who had been drawn from college students enrolled in a general psychology course) identical capsules containing either an inert placebo (milk sugar) or one of two drugs (5 mg dextroamphetamine or 2 grains caffeine) in a double-blind procedure. The findings were that 33.9 percent of males and 55.6 percent of females responded to the placebo. An inventory (the "General Attitude Variability Inventory," GAVI) was constructed, with test items concerning anxiety, religiousness, self-sufficiency, attitudes toward self, dominance, and dependency. Placebo reactors tended to score high on the GAVI and nonreactor subjects to score low. A year later, thirty males and thirty females from another introductory psychology class were selected on the basis of their high and low scores on the GAVI. These subjects were given both the drug and the placebo in a counterbalanced order, and these findings were that high scorers reacted significantly to the placebo, and low scorers did not react. Again, more females than males reacted, and out of all the items on the GAVI, those concerned with anxiety, self-sufficiency and dominance characterized the placebo reactors—that is, those persons who were subject to much anxiety, felt that they were insufficient in most situations, and felt they often seemed to be dominated by other people. The opposite held true for nonreactors.

Some similar personality variables were investigated by Gelfand, Gelfand, and Rardin (1965), whose experiment we encountered in the chapter on the use of placebos in studies of analgesia. The effects on placebo responsivity of subjects' self-esteem, social desirability, authoritarianism, and religious beliefs and behavior were studied in an experiment involving exposure of nonpatient subjects to ultrasonic stimulation, the administration of inert placebo, and then reexposure to ultrasonic stimulation. Thresholds and tolerance of induced pain were measured in both administrations. Both the religiosity scores and scores on social desirability were significantly related (positively) to pain tolerance in those subjects who reacted to the placebos, but no personality variable was related to pain threshold scores. This relationship of personality factors with tolerance but not with threshold measures supported the hypothesis that pain threshold is more highly loaded with physiological components than psychological components. This experiment was criticized previously because the subjects were not patients. The fact that some pain was involved here does, however, bring this particular experimental analogue a small step closer to the "real" placebo administration situation than is the case for the other experiments mentioned thus far in this chapter.

Linton and Langs (1962), whose study on placebo reactions was mentioned previously in this book (in the section on hallucinogenic drugs in chapter 3), divided their subjects (who were male professional actors) into strong and weak reactors to a tap-water placebo. The average of each subject's total scores for the two-hour, five-hour, and eight-hour questionnaire administrations was computed, and those above the median were considered strong placebo reactors and those below the median, weak ones. Seventy-three personality variables were used. These were derived from assessments of subjects made by staff members. Extensive psychological test and interview data were obtained, with no knowledge of subjects' behavior in the experiment. The areas of motives, defenses, thought processes, inner states, identity, and interpersonal behavior eventually yielded seventy-three variables. Strong and weak reactors differed on fourteen of these at the 0.05 level of significance. Strong reactors were characterized as bland and uncommunicative, with general passivity and passive resistance. They were suggestible and dependent on others to take the initiative, disorganized and unadaptive under stress, and had feelings of helplessness. They also showed what Linton and Langs called "loose thinking," with loose, vague, unclear concepts, and communication. Weak reactors (i.e., strong reactors lacked these) were characterized as having well-modulated affect and good temper and socially perceptive behavior. They often felt angry and impatient with themselves, showed goal striving in the face of frustration, were introspective and sensitive to minimal cues, and showed skillful problem analysis. They showed intellectualization and intellectuality, sought creative outlets, and showed sensitive, creative identity and philosophical concerns.

These variables represent four major areas of personality: On activity-passivity, the strong reactors tended to show greater passivity and suggestibility than weak reactors. They were more poorly defended. Weak reactors persisted in striving for their goals and redoubled their efforts when frustrated. Expression of affect differed in the two groups: The strong reactors showed a weak affect, and the weak reactors seemed to be good tempered, with well-modulated and flexible affect expressions. The two other groups of variables are closely related, according to Linton and Langs. Those variables most closely related to the strength of the placebo reaction indicated that "weak placebo reactors are more sensitive to both internal and external cues and conceive of themselves as sensitive. They are socially perceptive as well as self-examining; their impatience with themselves may reflect both self-doubt and the maintenance of high standards of achievement" (Linton and Langs 1962, p. 377). The variables dealing with intellectual functioning showed that weak placebo reactors saw themselves as intellectuals—that is, as being intellectually alert and curious. They functioned more effectively in intellectual tasks. Intellectualization tends to be used as a defense; "the context suggests that it is an appropriate and effective defense for them. The strong placebo reactors, in contrast, show thinking which is loose and vague and poorly communicated" (Linton and Langs 1962, p. 378).

The study by Linton and Langs was mentioned at this point because it is an interesting example of an experiment in which the use of nonpatient subjects *is* appropriate insofar as the "drug" used (LDS-25 placebo) is one that, at least in illicit usage, is frequently encountered in nonclinical situations. The ecological validity of the study, therefore, is somewhat higher than those we have encountered so far in this section, and the results of the study are more acceptable according to that criterion. In contrast, a study by Halm (1968), using college students as subjects, did not reveal significant differences between placebo reactors and nonreactors.

Halm (1968) conducted a study to investigate whether drug instructions generated appropriate mood changes and whether the cognitive control principle of field articulation accounted for individual differences in the observed placebo effect. The mean age of the college student subjects was 21, all subjects were male, and they were selected, not according to specifically designed question-naires, but rather the Group Embedded Figures Test. From a group of 122 students, Halm selected 20 field-dependent and 20 field-independent subjects for a total of 40. All 40 were given the Bass Social Acquiescence Scale prior to any treatment, and baseline measures in the Clyde Mood Scale were established, as well as baseline measures on nonspecific GSR. Subjects were then divided into two groups receiving different "drug" instructions accompanied by a liquid placebo. Twenty subjects received energizing instructions, and 20 tranquilizing instructions. Each group consisted of 10 field-dependent and 10 field-independent subjects. Following a 10-minute pause to simulate time necessary for drug effects, subjects were reevaluated on the Clyde Mood Scale and nonspecific GSR. The results showed that drug instructions did indeed operate to generate appropriate placebo effects when measured by mood changes in friendly, aggressive, sleepy, and unhappy mood factors. Nonspecific GSR was not sensitive to differences in drug instructions. The variables in which we are particularly interested here (i.e., those related to field articulation) did not, however, operate as expected in distinguishing placebo reactors from nonreac-tors. For mood change, field articulation was found to have, at best, a very restricted effect and to operate on an interactive basis with the magnitude of the placebo responses on friendly and sleepy mood factors and their respective baseline positions. This study also found that social acquiescence (as measured on the Bass Scale) did not correlate with field articulation, but it was associated with the magnitude of the placebo reaction for the sleepy mood factor. There was no relationship between the GSR and any of the other measures used.

The results of this investigation do not mean that personality differences between the placebo reactors and nonreactors did not exist, but merely that, if such differences did in fact exist, the particular measuring instruments used did not disclose them. If the subjects had been patients, knowing whether the Group Embedded Figures Test would have revealed differences in the scores of reactors and nonreactors, with the reactors being field dependent and the nonreactors field independent, would be interesting additional information. If such a relationship were to emerge, we would have additional evidence with which to stress the importance of the therapeutic milieu for meaningful research on the placebo effect, and the argument for using only patients as subjects would become more persuasive.

Using sixty nursing personnel volunteers, Guy (1967) carried out a study designed to determine the relationship of placebo proneness to environmental factors and personality traits: The subjects were randomly assigned to drug or placebo groups, and all subjects were "administered a test battery to measure pertinent personality variables" (p. 2138). (The contents of this test battery were not specified.) Placebo response was measured at intervals of zero, two, and twenty-four hours on the subjective level by critical flicker frequency, auditory RT, and a dynamometer task. This study is particularly interesting because, as a result of their professional activities, the subjects were all aware of the effects of the active drug, Thorazine, that was administered. Subjects were not told the nature of the drug, but guessed its identity according to their familiarity with its appearance. Another interesting aspect of the study is that the placebo employed was an active one: An equivalent dosage of Thorazine in capsule form. Subjects were told that the capsules contained a less potent drug than the tablets. Significant differences were shown when the effects of the tablet were compared to those of the capsule. These differences emerged on both the behavioral and autonomic levels. While the frequencies of symptoms reported under these two conditions did not differ significantly, the kinds of symptoms reported were different; all differences were in the direction predicted by the instructions minimizing the potency of the capsule. Also, the response curve on the dynamometer task obtained by subjects who had received the capsule was significantly lower than for those who had received the tablet. No pattern that would support the existence of an identifiable class of placebo reactor was revealed. However, on a less broad level of analysis, this study found that the general traits of neuroticism and introversion bore a significant relationship to placebo proneness, and neuroticism was also significantly correlated with pretreatment variability—that is, subjects who exhibited the greatest pre- and post- differences under baseline (no-treatment) conditions subsequently exhibited the greatest response to either drug or placebo. Guy concluded that placebo proneness in his subjects was significantly related to the level of emotional lability and to the magnitude of behavioral variation at pretreatment, rather than to a specific personality type.

Since Guy's (1967) experiment used a placebo that was an active drug, we might side-track for a moment here to note with interest that the fact is well-known that even active psychotropic drugs can produce widely differing effects in subjects of different personality types. For example, DiMascio and Rinkel (1963), in a paper presented at the Third World Congress of Psychiatry, Montreal, 1961, reported that "normal" subjects who reacted quite differently to two tranquilizing drugs (reserpine and phenyltoloxamine) possessed distinctive and contrasting personality types, as assessed on the basis of psychiatric interviews and the MMPI. On the MMPI, the "athletic" type scored low on *D*, high on *Ma*, low on *Si*, high on *Ess*, and low on the *MAS*. The "aesthetic" type scored high on *D*, low on *Ma*, high on *Si*, low on *Ess*, and high on *MAS*. Using the psychotomimetic drugs LSD-25, mescaline, and psilocybine, "athletic" persons generally reacted with marked euphoria and physiological disturbance, while the "aesthetic" types responded to the drugs predominantly with mental confusion and disruption of intellectual functioning. Individual variation in response to drugs is a fundamental characteristic of human subjects. In a paper presented at the Fourth World Congress of Psychiatry, Madrid, 1966, DiMascio (1968) mentioned that drug actions that are clinically useful can be noted in healthy people, that personality plays an important role in determining the total pattern of observed drug effect, and that paradoxical reactions to some tranquilizers can be predicted in some persons with specific personality patterns.

A study using the MMPI conducted by Kornetsky and Humphries (1957) also found drug-personality interactions, and Lasagna (1963), in a paper read at the Third World Congress of Psychiatry, reported a correlation between subjective responses after active drugs and the personality state of the subjects. Lasagna wrote that there is abundant evidence that on many occasions nondrug variables are *as* important, or more important, than the drug in contributing to the net "drug reaction." He saw the situation as being analogous to the growth of a plant: "Without a seed, there can be no plant, but there is also needed some soil, moisture, sunshine, etc. The size and nature of the plant is in part determined by the seed, to be sure, but to a large extent also by non-seed variables. For a gardener to overlook the latter and conceive of plant growth as an inevitable and totally predictable consequence of seed-planting is not only fallacious, but also often pragmatically disastrous. I suggest that we cultivate our psycho-pharmacologic gardens" (Lasagna 1963, p. 129). Thus we see that personality almost wrecks the determinism with which we might hope the mechanism of active agents to be imbued, and this is so to an even greater degree when we use placebos.

That factors in the "drug"-giving situation may even actually override personality type in responding to a placebo was demonstrated by Knowles and Lucas (1960) in a series of experiments under both "individual" and "group" conditions. All the subjects, who were students, were asked to report on the side effects of a new psychotropic drug that was actually a small white lactose tablet. In the "individual" condition, subjects assessed the effects of the tablet while seated alone in a room. In the "group" condition, subjects were seated together in groups of three. In two experiments carried out under the latter condition, there was a significant relationship between neuroticism, as measured on the Maudsley Personality Inventory, and the number of placebo side effects reported. As neuroticism increased, there was an increase in the number of "symptoms" reported after taking the placebo. Interestingly, these findings were in marked contrast with those of the two "individual" condition experiments, in which the correlation between neuroticism and the frequency of side effects was zero. Only when other influences (mainly social) were present, neuroticism was an important determinant of the placebo effect. We can therefore see that under group conditions of administration of medications (e.g., on a psychiatric ward), side effects from surrounding people might well be transmitted to suggestible neurotics. Some complex relationships with extroversion, as measured on the Maudsley Personality Inventory, were also reported. In the group experiments there was no overall relationship between placebo and extroversion, but in one of the "individual" experiments, there was a high positive correlation. In the second of these experiments, where the subjects were theology students, the relationship was not high and positive; in fact the introverted subjects showed the greatest placebo response. The high positive correlation was found in nursing students, and Knowles and Lucas (1960) suggested that theology students had little background knowledge of drugs and therefore reported on minor effects that would have been disregarded by the nurses. Introverts would be more meticulous in doing so; hence their greater placebo effect. An interesting comparison can be made of the effects of the knowledge of drug effects in this study and those in Guy's (1967) study, mentioned above, where subjects were also nurses.

Thorn (1962) administered the Taylor Manifest Anxiety Scale, the Maudsley Personality Inventory, and a symptom-measuring questionnaire to an experimental group of forty-five and a matched control group of twenty-four female undergraduates. Each subject was given the symptom questionnaire once a day for four days. These were the baseline measures. Each experimental subject was then given a one-grain red capsule of sugar crystals (presented as a new drug of unspecified nature and effects) once a day for four days and an hour later the symptom-measuring questionnaire. The control group filled in the questionnaire for the same time period of four days. Postexperimental inquiry revealed that only two subjects in the experimental group believed a placebo was being used. The placebo reaction score was the total frequency of response change shown to all items of the questionnaire by each subject when her preplacebo responses were compared to her responses while receiving placebo. Anxiety had a statistically significant correlation of +0.35 with reaction to the placebo, with highly anxious subjects reporting more symptoms both with and without placebo than did low anxiety subjects. In addition, a significant correlation of +0.30 was found between introversion and response to placebo. In

Thorn's (1962) view, these findings are "consistent with Eysenck's picture of the introverted neurotic or dysthymic, characterized by 'anxiety, reactive depression and/or obsession compulsion features.' It is suggested that subjects classified as prone to anxiety, depression and neurotic introverted tendencies react to placebo in the sense that such reactions are overt manifestations of anxiety" (p. 6). Despite the fact that the correlations given were significant, they were quite low and accounted for only 12.25 percent of the variance in the case of the anxiety measures and 9 percent in the case of the introversion measure. There is some relationship, to be sure, but it is lower than one would want before one asserts that anxiety and introversion are important determinants, in this experiment, of the placebo effect.

Studies in which the subjects were patients. The only report that I have been able to locate in which the personality of the placebo reactor in "psychopharmacological" (i.e., placebo) treatment was measured in *patients* by using nonprojective tests was presented by Rickels (1968b) at the Fourth World Congress of Psychiatry in Madrid, 1966. The experimental design and the statistics used were, unfortunately, not mentioned in the article. The relationship of pretreatment scores of a number of selected personality variables to indices of improvement after four weeks of treatment with antianxiety drugs (meprobamate or chlordiazepoxide) or placebo was assessed. More patients of low verbal intelligence improved on placebo than did those of high verbal intelligence. More patients showing low anxiety (Taylor MAS) improved than did those of high anxiety. Placebo patients who improved showed a higher self-rating of potency or adequacy (semantic differential) than those who did not improve. These differences were significant below the 0.05 level.

The Use of Projective Personality Instruments in Assessing the Personality of Placebo Reactors

The number of studies in this area is even more sparse than that using nonprojective personality tests. Despite the controversy over the validity of projective tests, the clinicians who use them seem to agree that they can be a useful source of data. Thus, before taking the stance that projective tests are unreliable, invalid, and rather useless remnants of a less sophisticated psychometric era, one should at least look at the studies in which they have been used. The purpose of this section is to review the literature on investigations of the personality of the placebo reactor and not to sharpen the swords of one particular viewpoint of what should constitute psychological assessment against those of another.

An early study, which has become a frequently cited classic of the placebo literature, was published by Lasagna, Mosteller, von Felsinger, and Beecher

(1954). The subjects were postoperative patients on the general surgical, urological, orthopedic, and gynecological wards of a general hospital. The time of observation was the period after surgery—that is, starting as soon as relief of pain became necessary and ending with the cessation of the need for narcotics. Postoperative pain for which morphine or a similar narcotic was ordered by the house staff was considered satisfactory for study. The subjects were aged seventeen to seventy-five.

Pain relief was studied in two main categories: first, steady wound pain while lying quietly in bed and, second, all other types of pain. A medication was considered to have produced relief when the patient indicated significant (over 50 percent) alleviation of pain at forty-five and again at ninety minutes after injection, and these responses were elicited by technicians unaware of the nature of the medication employed. The study was conducted in two phases. In phase I, sixty-nine patients were studied. For every six active medications each patient received, one dose was a placebo (1 ml saline solution). The other five were doses of morphine phosphate (10 mk/kg). The order of administration was randomized, so that some patients received the placebo first, some second, and so on. In phase II, ninety-three patients were studied. Placebo and morphine doses were alternated in each patient, and the starting dose (i.e., placebo or morphine) was alternated from patient to patient. From the ninety-three patients in phase II, twenty-four were chosen because they had responded in consistent fashion to doses of placebo: Eleven of these always obtained pain relief, and thirteen always failed to experience pain relief. In addition, three other patients were chosen because they were considered nonreactors on the basis of failing on most occasions (four of five, five of six, and seven of eight responses, respectively) to obtain pain relief from placebo. An important note here is that these twenty-seven patients represented a screened sample: Only responses to steady severe wound pain were considered, and for every placebo dose that produced relief, a return of pain was required in order to eliminate the possibility that the pain had subsided spontaneously.

Consistent reactors and nonreactors were employed in the hope that such a procedure would heighten the contrast between such groups. Psychological data were obtained by psychologists and technicians who were unaware of the nature of the placebo responses. (The authors did not explicitly state, however, to what extent the *whole* study could be considered to be double-blind.) The psychological data consisted of an interview; questionnaires filled out by the nurses concerning patients' personality, social relationships, and hospital course; a Rorschach test; a TAT; and an estimation of IQ based on the vocabulary subtest of the Wechsler-Bellevue Scale. The interview, Rorschach, TAT, and WAIS subtest were all administered at the end of the hospital stay, just prior to discharge.

Regarding pain relief, the trend in both phases was for less pain relief to occur, the greater the number of placebo doses administered over time. This finding suggests that, like morphine, doses of placebo were less effective in patients who received many doses of medication and whose pain was of long duration. In phase II, 55 percent of the patients did not show a consistent response to placebo, 14 percent were consistent reactors, and 31 percent were not placebo reactors. The WAIS data revealed no intelligence differences between reactors and nonreactors, and even though the TAT was used, no data for this test were given (which does not mean that we can assume that no significant differences between reactors and nonreactors on the TAT measures used were found). The results in which we are most interested here did, however, show some extremely striking differences between reactors and nonreactors on the basis of data obtained from the Rorschach and the interviews.

First of all, let us examine the interview material. The investigators found that the reactors perceived the discomfort of the pain and of the postoperative period to be less severe than did the nonreactors and that all the reactors considered the hospital care "wonderful," while only 25 percent of the nonreactors felt this way. In addition, the following characterized the placebo reactors: They tended to ask less frequently for medications; were more cooperative with the nursing staff; had, in the case of females, more severe menstrual pain (and took medications for such pain); tended to have more somatic symptoms ("nervous stomach," diarrhea, headache) during periods of stress; used more cathartics and aspirin-type drugs; were more emotionally expressive in the testing situation and spoke more freely; said that they "liked everyone"; had had less formal education; and were more frequent church goers than the nonreactors.

On Rorschach test, the investigators found that six signs were common to 60 percent of the reactor group, while none of the nonreactors was so characterized (only one nonreactor had as many as four signs). The six signs were: (1) more than one "insides" response; (2) $\Sigma C > M$; (3) A% below 50%; (4) $CF > FC$; (5) more than two "anxiety" responses; (6) less than two "hostility" responses. Submitting the differential distribution of the reactors and nonreactors who had all six signs to Fisher's exact test showed significance at less than the 0.01 level, and a test of the distribution of the groups based on any four signs also gave this probability value. (The Rorschach scoring and interpretation were based primarily on the system of Kelley and Klopfer.)

In contrast to the nonreactors, the reactors were more productive of responses, more anxious, more self-centered and preoccupied with internal bodily processes, and more emotionally labile. They were persons who seemed more dependent on outside stimulation than on their own mental processes, which tended to be less mature than in the case of nonreactors. In general, the reactors were persons whose instinctive needs were greater and whose control over the social expression of these needs was less strongly defined and developed than in the nonreactors. While they were more anxious and dependent, the fact that they were also more labile and outwardly oriented might enable them to relieve this anxiety and tension more easily than nonreactors might. Over a period of time, they might appear less anxious because of their ability to "drain off the tension," as evidenced by the fact that in interviews they were found to be more talkative than the nonreactors. According to the authors, the most striking characteristic of the reactors was the great frequency of responses dealing with the abdominal and pelvic viscera. The high incidence of these responses, and their extremely poor form level, would be considered definitely pathological except for the fact that a certain amount of preoccupation with one's bodily processes may be expected in a hospital setting. The reactor group produced many more such responses than the nonreactors.

This study is one of the few that presents fairly detailed characteristics of the nonreactors. They did not, by contrast to the reactors, present a "normal" picture: While showing less deviation than the reactors, they were far more rigid and emotionally controlled than the average person for their ages and back-grounds. Since the pressures and tensions of the hospital situation presumably accentuated the protective and defensive mechanisms of their personalities, the rigidity of the nonreactors might well have been an expression of their defense mechanisms in a stressful situation.

Several criticisms can be made of this study. First of all, we noticed earlier that only 14 percent of the patients reacted consistently to the placebo. This percentage was quite low when compared with the percentage who were inconsistent reactors (55 percent) and the percentage (31 percent) who did not react favorably to the placebo. Such a small percentage is perhaps a bit low to suggest that the same patients would react in the same way to placebos under different conditions and that the picture that emerged is a "true" one of the personality of such persons.

Second, an interesting criticism was made by Trouton (1957) who stated that, since all the reactors were found by Lasagna et al. to have been "veritable pillar(s) of the church, attending services with regularity and being greatly interested and active in church affairs," possibly they entered the hospital more prepared and more able to tolerate pain uncomplainingly. Christianity, according to Trouton, is apt at least in theory to foster a peculiar and "unbiological" attitude of acceptance of pain and suffering. Thus, since 72 percent of the reactors, as compared with 19 percent of the nonreactors, were said to minimize postoperative pain, Lasagna et al. appear to depend for their measurement of pain on complaints of people who, both in theory and in practice, are relatively uncomplaining. Further supporting this objection are the findings that the reactors asked for medication less frequently, were more cooperative, and had less formal education. However, nurses said that they had the impression that these patients had less severe pain, but the nurses could only observe the overt *reactions* to the pain, which would, of course, be less according to the view put forward here. These patients gave a history of more somatic symptoms under stress, said that they had a greater tendency to use aspirins and cathartics, and at the interview were more "weepy" and more talkative. The P of these differences ranges from 0.10 or less to 0.001. "It would be of interest to know how frequently the injections of morphine and of the placebo were accompanied by nausea; if the incidence should prove higher in the non-reactor group, this would support the interpretation given above (Trouton 1957, p. 348)."

As was pointed out earlier in this chapter, the administration of the personality assessment devices should be carried out prior to treatment. In this experiment, personality was assessed during the patients' convalescent phase, at which time they might not have been in their "normal" psychological state. While one could make a case for the importance of the measurement of state variables here, trait variables should not be neglected in this way, particularly if one wishes to develop guidelines for the use of placebos in particular situations with particular patients. Another criticism of the experiment is that since there was no objective measure of the drug effect or of the pain, daily alterations could not be recorded.

We have already encountered, in the section on placebo effects in studies of LSD-25, the study by Abramson, Jarvik, Levine, Kaufman, and Hirsch (1955), in which some subjects received the active drug, LSD-25, while others received placebos. On the basis of a symptom questionnaire, subjects were divided into high and low symptom groups. The number of subjects in each group was extremely small ($n = 6$), but significant differences in certain Rorschach variables were found when analyzing their protocols (the test had been administered before treatment). The investigators (using Klopfer's system) found that the high symptom group scored higher on D, S, M, m, FC, CF, C, F%, H+A, Hd+Ad, and W:M than the low symptom group, who scored higher on W, Dd, FM, c, C', F+%, new F+%, M:C, FM+m, C+C, R8-10%, and M:FM than did the high symptom group.

The investigators also obtained data on the WAIS and on the basis of this test and the Rorschach responses, found that the low responders tended to be primarily action oriented in their adaptive efforts, while those in the high response group tended to be ideationally oriented. Only some subtests (Arithmetic and Block Design) showed significant differences between the groups on the WAIS. However, the suggested difference was present in eight out of ten subtests, and within this framework, the authors suggested that those who performed better on a verbal level appeared to be more suggestible and hence showed a greater placebo response. Those in the low group tended, as suggested by their responses on the Rorschach, to be more stereotyped in their thinking and emphasized the popular and conventional modes of responding.

More recently, Rickels (1968b) reported the following Rorschach data in a study discussed previously in this chapter, but gave no details of the procedure of the study, which concerned relationships between a number of selected personality variables and indices of improvement after treatment with antianxiety drugs (meprobamate or chlordiazepoxide) or placebo. The relationship between compliance, as measured on the Rorschach test, and indices of improvement after treatment with the drugs or placebo were assessed. After four weeks of treatment, 83 percent of the improved drug patients, and only 54 percent of the improved placebo patients, were found to show high compliance. The percentage of improved drug patients and placebo patients showing low compliance was quite close: 56 percent and 58 percent, respectively. The differences between the high compliance patients on drugs and placebo were statistically significant at the 5 percent level, as were those between the high compliance and low compliance patients on drugs. "Compliance, interestingly, produced its primary effect on drug patients; from this one may hypothesize that even minimal, yet beneficial, drug effects (e.g., sedation or relaxation) may serve as a catalyst for a good doctor-patient relationship in the more compliant patient, resulting in more systematic improvement" (Rickels 1968b, p. 11).

Shapiro, Wilensky, and Struening (1968), whose experiment on a placebo effect using a placebo test was reviewed in chapter 6, found that various projective measures (F scale, TAT, Rorschach M, EM, Ec, DL) showed statistically significant differences between reactors and nonreactors, depending on the method of scoring used. According to Shapiro et al. (1968), ". . . psychological variables indicated that the main difference was between reactors in general, without regard to direction, and nonreactors. For method B, there are very few differences between positive and negative reactors. But with total count of placebo responses (Method A), only [one] variable was statistically significant for both positive and negative reactors [the Rorschach EM] . . . . The percent response (Method C) had another pattern. Most of the significant differences occurred with neutrals and negatives. The patterns of correlation . . . indicated that the placebo response is complicated; different patterns emerge with different methods of treatment" (p. 125).

The authors interpreted the results of these tests as indicating that negative reactors had more available inner fantasy, relied on inner stimulation, and were less dependent on the environment. Positive reactors relied on environment more than on inner processes. Positive reactors tend to be field dependent and rely on outer stimuli (e.g., the setting and placebo test procedure probably stimulated cues for placebo responses), while negative reactors tended to ignore the field and rely on inner stimuli, and neutral reactors tended to deny both outer and inner stimuli.

We now turn to the next section on the personality of the placebo reactor and attempt to see whether, given additional data, some of the findings mentioned thus far can be more cohesively explained.

*Suggestibility, Acquiescence, Hypnosis, and
the Placebo Reactor*

We have seen that a commonly advanced explanation of the placebo effect is one vaguely involving the subject's "suggestibility." This word, however, means nothing without specifying exactly which variables are thought to be involved, and such definition has seldom been provided. One cannot deny that some (albeit too few) investigators have attempted to find out what suggestion is and where it is operative (e.g., in patient, therapist, situational, and interactional variables) but the analyses are often too molar for anything meaningful to emerge.

"Suggestion," having acquired official status, is unfortunately beginning to play in many quarters the part of a wet blanket upon investigation, being used to fend off all inquiry into the varying susceptibilities of individual cases. "Suggestion" is only another name for the power of ideas, so far as they prove efficacious over belief and conduct. Ideas efficacious at some times and in some surroundings are not so at other times and elsewhere . . . the mere waving of the word "suggestion" as if it were a banner gives no light.

These words were not written yesterday by a modern experimental psychologist, but came from the pen of the great William James, some seventy-five years ago (*The Varieties of Religious Experience*, 1901). In viewing all of James' points, we can see that things are not much different now from what they were seventy-five years ago. Even the problem of "the varying susceptibilities of individual cases" has not been solved: There are many tests of suggestibility, each of which can differentiate between subjects, but the comparison of different studies and different situations is made very difficult by the fact that so many different tests are used and the correlations between these tests themselves are significantly low (and even, in some cases, negative!).

Some other problems with tests of suggestibility were pointed out by Abramson, Jarvik, Levine, Kaufman, and Hirsch (1955). When questionnaires are used, the number of positive responses made is partly a function of the questions asked. Also, a questionnaire used as an instrument for measuring suggestibility can be problematical in that the response threshold of subjects is not determined. Equally suggestible subjects who experience the same severity of a symptom may differ in the degree of change which must be present before responding with a symptom. In addition, when more than one subject is tested (e.g., dyads or groups being tested together), responses of subjects can influence the responses of the placebo subject in whom we are particularly interested here. Because of the variable effects found under different circumstances, observations concerning subjects who are classified as "high" or "low" regarding their suggestibility can be applied only in the specific settings under consideration and cannot legitimately be used as "labels" for the subjects when they are placed in other settings.

Several studies have been carried out in an attempt to verify the widely hypothesized relationships between placebo responsiveness and either suggestibility or susceptibility to hypnosis or both suggestibility *and* susceptibility to hypnosis. While this book is not really the place to enter into a discussion of the validity of the concept of hypnosis as a state of the organism, we cannot reasonably deal with any aspects related to this phenomenon without making at least brief mention of the fact that a controversy, which is sometimes quite a heated one, exists about whether we have good grounds for dismissing hypnosis as a "nothing but . . ." phenomenon (e.g., Barber 1969) or whether we still have good reason for adopting the stance that hypnosis is a state (e.g., Tellegen 1970) to be investigated as such. The essence of Barber's approach is that the hypnotic induction process is unnecessary for the appearance of any of the hypnotic trance phenomena, and in a variety of studies, he has attempted to show that little difference appears in the performance of subjects given instructions in the trance state and those given waking suggestions. Barber's research also attempts to show that there is nothing new even in the hypnotic trance: Any phenomenon, even physiological events, may be performed as well by subjects given suggestions in the waking state as those given suggestions during trance. Barber's pursuit of his essentially debunking research has been very rigorous, and he always uses the words "hypnosis," "hypnotic," and so forth in quotation marks.

How does this information help us in our search for the personality of the placebo responder? Although the attempt to assess the relationship of suggestibility to other personality variables has not been made in all the studies to be presented here, I would like to put forward the notion that both suggestibility and hypnotizability could possibly be "phenotypic" (if that word may be used in this context) of some "genotypic" characteristics, and further work on the relationship of these factors, both to one another and to placebo responsiveness, could perhaps—provided that their molarity were reduced by more sophisticated analysis—give us some clues on which to base future research strategies in this area. A brief note should also be added here that these comments on suggestibility and hypnosis have been included as a prologue of caution akin to well-ground spectacles to be worn when reading about any research in this area. Far too few investigators have either acknowledged, or have seemingly even been aware of, the difficulties with which their supposed "insight" into these relationships are fraught. Let us first examine studies on suggestibility and placebo responsiveness.

Suggestibility. An important consideration in this problem-laden area is that suggestibility is not a unitary characteristic. The old classification by Eysenck and Furneaux (1945; see also Claridge 1972, p. 37) posited that suggestibility consists of two unrelated components: primary and secondary suggestibility. Primary suggestibility refers to the tendency to react to suggestion with motor movements, for example, on the Body Sway Test. Secondary suggestibility refers to the induction of feelings or perceptions in the subject. A major review by Evans (1967) on suggestibility in the normal waking state stated that Eysenck's classification cannot be justified either on the basis of the original data presented to support it or from subsequent research. Evans showed that three types of suggestibility now seem identifiable. The first of these, primary suggestibility, involves passive (motor) suggestions. In these, the subject does not play an overt active role in producing the movement but rather passively awaits its occurrence. The second is challenge suggestibility, which consists of two components: a suggested inhibition of movement followed by a challenge to overcome the inhibited response (e.g., suggesting that the subject cannot bend his or her arm and then testing the inhibited movement by a challenge to overcome the induced rigidity). The third type of suggestibility is imagery (sensory) suggestibility, for example, the Heat Illusion Test, in which subjects report when they first feel warmth in an object held in their hands or to their foreheads and continue to report that they experience heat as the experimenter increases a (nonexistent) current on successive trials. These three types of suggestibility warrant further independent investigation.

Eysenck's classification does not make clear whether the placebo effect may involve mainly primary suggestibility or mainly secondary suggestibility, or whether it is a combination of the two. When questionnaires of suggestibility are used, they almost universally involve secondary suggestibility. Using Evans' classification makes it likely that any of the three could be involved, with most questionnaires presumably tapping sensory/imagery suggestibility. Classification on this basis is, however, difficult since most of the suggestibility tests have previously been classified as belonging to one or the other Eysenckian category.

A study by Steinbook, Jones, and Ainslie (1965) involved the relationship between primary suggestibility and the placebo effect. Scores on the Press Test were obtained, and then twenty psychiatric outpatients were treated with a placebo for two weeks. Half of the group remained on the placebo therapy for another four weeks. A psychiatrist evaluated each patient's symptoms at each of seven visits. Although suggestibility scores on the Press Test were found to be positively correlated ($r = +0.71$) with the decline in the number severity of presenting symptoms in the first two weeks, this correlation was much weaker at the end of therapy. The correlation between the suggestibility scores and the increase in "subsequent symptoms" was negative and was attributed by the authors to a generalization of the therapeutic effect or a manifestation of disapproval in the nonsuggestible patients. The thought did not seem to occur to the investigators that such patients might really have had a remission in posttherapy symptoms. Also, Evans (1967) has pointed out that this result is equivocal because of the impossibility of determining whether suggestibility is correlated with the initial frequency of presenting symptoms and hence is spuriously correlated with the immediate decrease of presenting symptoms (i.e., no correlation was reported between suggestibility and the number of symptoms initially reported).

Measuring suggestibility and then seeing how this is related to placebo responsivity is not, as Duke (1964) found, an easy task. He attempted to measure placebo reactivity with tests of suggestibility in aging residents of a nursing home who were on placebo therapy for insomnia. However, since the questionnaire to measure placebo reactivity was not validated (so that the reported placebo reactivity may not actually be a measure of the experienced reactivity) and, moreover, since the finding that placebo reactivity correlated only low (but positively) with primary suggestibility (in the Eysenckian sense) and not with secondary suggestibility, we should be very cautious in accepting the results of this study.

Evans (1967) reviewed a number of other studies on the placebo effect and suggestibility, all of which were conducted before 1967. Significant relationships only seemed to emerge when the subjects were patients. Evans cited a study by Imber, Frank, Nash, Gliedman, and Stone (1956), in which the investigators found that body sway suggestibility is greater in those patients who remain in psychotherapy than in those who drop out. This finding may explain the discrepancy apparently existing between clinical findings, which are positive, and experimental findings, which are negative, for a relationship between suggestibility and placebo. Possibly, mechanisms are operative in therapy that are *quote* "common to both suggestibility and placebo responsiveness which lead to an apparent statistical relationship between suggestibility and placebo responsiveness in a patient-therapist situation, but when this common therapeutic factor does not exist in a subject-experimenter context, the statistical association is not found" (Evans 1967, p. 127). This sort of evidence provides additional support for the recurrent argument made in this book regarding ecological validity and placebo experiments.

Acquiescence. A similar trait to suggestibility, acquiescence, has recently been examined in placebo reactors, and, as we shall see, the literature is impressive in content and formidable in amount. Acquiescence is a kind of "yea saying"—that is, a tendency to respond in ways that are pleasing or acceptable to others. It often occurs in the completion of personality and other inventories as a response bias toward giving the answer "yes" indiscriminately to questions irrespective of their content. An experiment by Fisher and Fisher (1963) gave some evidence that in certain situations a tendency toward acquiescence is more pronounced in placebo reactors than in nonreactors. Subjects were asked to report any effects they noted after taking what they were told was a harmless but pharmacologically active pill, which was actually a placebo. An "electrode" (actually a sham one) was attached to each subject's fingertip and wired to a polygraph recording device. This procedure reinforced the subjects' believing that the physiological effects of an active drug were being studied. Each subject was periodically asked whether any changes had been noticed. After ten minutes each was told that the time of the maximum effect of the pill was approaching. Subjects reported many physical symptoms such as stomach pain and itchy skin. They were then asked to complete a questionnaire measuring acquiescence, and the investigators found that those who were highly acquiescent also reported a significantly greater frequency of side effects to the placebo. Ideally, the acquiescence questionnaire should have been administered before the treatment in order to avoid the possible influence of during-treatment variables on the results.

An article on placebo effects, response set, and acquiescence was presented by Pichot and Perse (1968) at the Fourth World Congress of Psychiatry, Madrid, 1966. The purpose of the paper was to present the hypothesis that there exists a correlation between the placebo effect and response set, together with some confirming evidence. Pichot and Perse showed how both response set and the placebo effect had been considered artifacts for a long time, with placebo effects making difficult the evaluation of efficacy in drug research and response set being of interest only insofar as its role as an invalidator of personality questionnaire results was concerned. However, the recognition of the placebo effect led to the use of the double-blind technique and gave impetus to a host of research. Similarly, response set became recognized as something considerably different from mere artifact with the publication of *The Authoritarian Personality* by Adorno et al. (1950), "and the criticisms of this work, which were based on the observation that the *F*-scale items gave one point for authoritarianism uniquely for the true responses, opened the controversy by suggesting that the score for authoritarianism was in reality only an index of acquiescence" (Pichot and Perse 1968, p. 51). The authors also mentioned a review in which Damarin and Messick (1965) examined the concepts and evidence concerning the psychological significance of response set and the possibility of relations between these attitudes and a number of other, independently measured personality characteristics. "Indeed, if response set in questionnaire responses is a function of basic personality characteristics, then these same characteristics would tend to affect biases in other situations" (Pichot and Perse 1968, p. 51). A parallel exists between the nature and determinants of the placebo effect and response set. We have already seen, in this book, that a point of contention in studies of the placebo effect is the existence of a reaction tendency independent of the particular circumstances that results in a definition of a class of identifiable, consistent placebo reactors. But an examination of the evidence derived from experimental studies leads to the adoption of a position that—in considering the type of subjects studied (patients or not), type of symptoms affected by therapy, and so forth—is more defined: A reaction to the administration of a placebo is seen as a behavior resulting from the interaction of both general factors (reactivity to the placebo) and specified ones (situation specific). In looking at particular response sets, "there are some indications that a single general expectational attitude has to be present. Such expectational attitude seems specific in function to the particular material to which it is applied" (Pichot and Perse 1968, p. 52). Thus the historical and conceptual similarities between the placebo effect and response set suggest that a strong relationship exists between the two phenomena, with a close analogy existing between acquiescence and the placebo effect, and negation and the nocebo effect.

The hypothesis of Pichot and Perse was that the placebo effect (or nocebo effect) is at least partially determined by the attitude of acquiescence (or negation) as it can be measured in personality questionnaires. The instruments used were the First Factor Scale (or Factor A Scale), constructed by Welsh (1956) from factor analyses of the MMPI, and Fricke's (1957) Response Bias Scale, constructed by selecting the sixty-three most controversial items of the MMPI. These were items to which "normal" subjects answer "true" or "false" about an equal number of times, with the number of "true" responses being used as the measure of acquiescence. Two independent experiments were conducted.

The first experiment involved 111 volunteer, male medical students, who were administered the group form of the MMPI and later took a placebo that was presented, under neutral conditions, as an experimental therapeutic product. The next morning all subjects completed a nine-item questionnaire concerning the effects experienced, and sixteen subjects who answered "yes" to a question on unusual fatigue prior to the experiment were eliminated, as were seventeen subjects who did not follow the experimental design. The four questions on which a subject could obtain a score of −1 (unfavorable effect), 0 (no effect), and +1 (favorable effect) concerned intellectual ability, intellectual fatigability, physical fatigability, and affective state. This score could vary from −4 to +4. Four questions concerned the presence or absence of these side effects: anxiety, motor tension, palpitations, and sleep disturbance. The results showed that 38 percent of all subjects reacted to the placebo with identical frequencies of positive and nocebo effects (19 percent). These identical frequencies may, according to the investigators, have been partially due to the neutral nature of their instructions. The responses of the seventy-eight subjects fell into three groups: positive response to placebo, no response to placebo, and nocebo response.

In the second experiment, fifty-three physicians who had taken the MMPI were asked to assist in a study seeking to determine precisely, under placebo control, the value of a new drug. Four identical envelopes, each labeled either week 1, 2, 3, or 4 and each containing seven capsules, were given to the subjects, who were informed that certain envelopes contained the experimental product and others, possibly the placebo. The subjects were required to indicate which weeks they believed that they received placebo and which weeks they had noticed the stimulating or tranquilizing effect of the new drug. The active drug was Librium (chlordiazepoxide), while the other capsules contained identically appearing and analogous-tasting placebo. The results fell into three groups: one group in which subjects responded to the placebo, one in which they did not, and a third group of subjects who correctly identified the placebo and the active drug and were excluded from future analysis. The second study was different from the first because the medication was administered for four weeks instead of one day, and subjects knew they were taking either an active drug or a placebo. The nonresponding group was therefore considered by the authors to have shown a nocebo effect as indicated by their lack of reaction to the active drug, as if they had adopted an attitude of negation sufficiently strong to counter the effects of the Librium.

The relationships between the results of both experiments and the acquiescence scores (using the Welsh and Fricke Scales) was as follows: first, a general responsiveness to placebo, independent of the situation and consequently relatively stable, does in fact exist and, second, that "the attitude of acquiescence is at least relatively independent of the contextual material. In our study the attitude describing the style of response to a personality questionnaire permits the prediction of an attitude of acquiescence or negation *vis à vis* the situation created by taking a placebo. These conclusions invite the study of the differential role that the several varieties of response sets may have on the appearance of placebo effects" (Pichot and Perse 1968, p. 57).

The results of the first experiment seem acceptable enough, apart from the objection raised earlier about the subjects (nonpatients) and hence the ecological validity of the experiment. However, in the second experiment, Pichot and Perse considered the nonresponding group to have shown a *nocebo* effect as indicated by their *lack of reaction* to the drug (Librium), as if they had adopted an attitude of negation sufficiently strong to counter the effects of the Librium. The investigators may not have been justified in making this assertion, since no response either to placebo or to an active drug is simply that (i.e., no response) and not a nocebo effect. Thus, the inference that an attitude of negation was involved is unfounded. The investigators, in addition, did not specify how they knew that the third group in the second experiment identified correctly both the placebo and the active drug (e.g., what reactions did subjects report in each treatment?), nor why such subjects were excluded from further analysis since they might have shown a distinctive pattern of response on the acquiescence measures, which should not, a priori, have been ruled out. Since, in addition, the order of administration of Librium and placebo in the second experiment was not specified and the percentage of the four-week period devoted to either placebo or Librium was not stated, the findings of that experiment and in particular its theoretical implications are not justified by the procedure.

An experiment that more strongly supports the relationship of acquiescence to the placebo effect was reported by McNair, Kahn, Droppleman, and Fisher (1968), also at the Fourth World Congress of Psychiatry, Madrid, 1966. McNair et al. studied patient acquiescence in a two-week double-blind comparison of diazepam versus placebo, with patients randomly assigned both to the medication and to the treating doctors. All patients were new admissions to a psychiatric clinic; forty-nine women and twenty men (mean age twenty-nine and of average education, including some college) completed the study. Measures on various predictors, including the Bass Scale and pretreatment criterion baselines, were taken immediately prior to the first interview, and the criterion measures (including mood measures, symptom distress measures, a measure of target symptoms, and improvement ratings) were repeated prior to the second and third treatment sessions. During the interviews, treating doctors elicited principal complaints, followed a brief routine for prescribing medication, and limited each of the three weekly contacts to a thirty-minute maximum. They recorded their observations and criterion ratings immediately after each visit. One research psychiatrist made the many decisions necessary to ensure patients' welfare, observed all interviews, interviewed each patient after the third interview with the treating doctor, and at this time, rated change on several criteria. Equal numbers of identically appearing tablets were prescribed to both medication groups, with the diazepam dosage being one 5 mg tablet t.i.d. When the study had been run, the median acquiescence score for the whole sample was calculated. Acquiescers were classified by the scores above this median, while nonacquiescers fell below it. The results, computed on the basis of a 2 x 2 analysis of either variance or covariance concerning interactions between acquiescence and medication, revealed that patient response to medication appeared to depend on level of acquiescence—that is, the relationship of acquiescence to outcome depended very much on the type of medication received. The investigators presented three sources of evidence, each of which sheds a somewhat different light on this outcome pattern: interactions after one week of treatment, interactions after two weeks of treatment, and interactions in a specific subset of patients.

In considering patient target symptoms (representing the patient's distress scores on the three complaints each had identified prior to treatment as major problems), the interaction was of borderline significance, with drug effectiveness appearing to depend on level of acquiescence. After one week of treatment, nonacquiescers showed a difference in favor of the drug. When only the low acquiescers were considered, the drug versus placebo mean difference was significant. Also, after one week of treatment, acquiescers on drug improved about the same as acquiescers on placebo. A similar pattern was shown on the tension-anxiety mood factor (from the Psychiatric Outpatient Mood Scales) and patient global improvement ratings as related to acquiescence. Acquiescers showed no difference between drug and placebo. "On all three criteria, it looked as though non-acquiescers were discriminating both medications and responded more favorably to the drug. Acquiescers appeared to respond about equally to drug and placebo. This failure to discriminate appeared to result from their very favorable response to placebo rather than a failure to improve with the drug" (McNair et al. 1968, p. 66).

After two weeks of treatment, the relationship of the tension-anxiety measures and acquiescence showed a crossover interaction: Nonacquiescers responded more favorably to diazepam, and acquiescers showed a more favorable response to placebo. On nearly every patient criterion measure, the same significant crossover interaction occurred. Nonacquiescers reacted more favorably to drug than placebo, and on several criteria acquiescers on placebo reported more improvement than nonacquiescers on drug. "In nearly every case, high acquiescers on drug showed less improvement than any other subgroup. In fact, on most criteria they reported either no change or a worsening of problems as compared with their pretreatment status. They were the only subgroup that did not show significant prepost improvement during the two weeks of the experiment" (McNair et al. 1968, p. 65).

A specific subset of patients was chosen in an attempt to provide additional control for the post hoc classification of patients. Five pairs (one receiving drug, one placebo) of female patients who were acquiescers and four pairs who were not were compared. Each pair had been treated by the same doctor, and each was comparable in acquiescence score. Two-way analyses of variance on the patient criterion scores for this subsample of eighteen patients yielded even more extensive examples of the crossover interaction on nearly all the improvement criteria than did the total sample of sixty patients.

Earlier in this chapter, we looked briefly at an experiment by Fisher and Fisher (1963). The placebo slopes in the figures given for the experiment by McNair et al. (1968) replicate those findings. In the absence of a no-medication control group, however, we cannot conclusively infer that acquiescers show more placebo effect than nonacquiescers. Even though, as McNair et al. point out, acquiescence scores could relate to the nature and prognosis of the illness and might imply differential improvement rates even if no placebo had been given, clearly, "acquiescers on placebo report so much improvement that a minor tranquilizer probably would have little chance of surpassing such an effect" (p. 68). The investigators also found that acquiescers reported considerably more somatic distress at the beginning of treatment and focused more on somatic issues in the interviews. Placebos led to reports of marked improvement in both somatic complaints and other areas. Paradoxically, tranquilizers did not have this effect.

Perhaps the acquiescers were simply responding to the demand characteristics of the situation, but "much evidence from this study and prior research suggests that acquiescers are likely to be rather thoughtless, nondiscriminating individuals, rather than compliant conformers" (McNair et al. 1968, p. 71). In fact, there was no independent evidence that acquiescers were more compliant or conforming to the research procedures. They were no more likely than nonacquiescers to take their medication as prescribed, and they were also somewhat more likely to omit test items, especially those involving self-description. Their adverse responses to the drug could have shown several things: unthinking, invalid, and unreliable test taking and verbal reporting. Sampling error may also have been operative. "Another possibility is that acquiescers respond with exaggerated, diffuse and, hence, nondiscriminating concern to whatever somatic cues are produced by the drug" (McNair et al., 1968, p. 71).

This study is, perhaps, one of the best designed and most carefully presented in the rather large volume of the placebo literature. The results were presented here in some detail not only because the study has not (as far as I am aware) been fully reviewed anywhere else, but also because the series of steps reads like an elegant investigation in which we ultimately have before us an excellent picture of our quarry.

Further evidence in the role of acquiescence in the placebo effect was presented by Fast and Fisher (1971) in an experiment concerning the role of body attitudes and acquiescence in epinephrine and placebo effects. Although the main details of the study are not immediately relevant to our discussion, three subsidiary hypotheses investigated in the study are of importance here. In an earlier experiment (Fisher and Fisher 1964), one of the authors had found that in "normal" subjects, degree of acquiescence was positively correlated with degree of placebo response, and this result was anticipated to be replicated in the second study (Fast and Fisher 1971). The authors cited the findings of a number of studies by McNair et al. (one of which we have just examined above) that improvement in psychiatric patients in response to a placebo correlated positively with their degree of acquiescence, and improvement in response to a real drug (diazepam) was negatively correlated to a degree of acquiescence. Highly acquiescent patients improved least on drug and most on placebo. In addition, since highly acquiescent patients were more likely to be somatic complainers and to be more easily aroused, McNair and his colleagues conjectured that highly acquiescent patients found a real drug to be more disturbing because of the somatic changes it produced. A placebo, in contrast, could arouse expectations of improvement but no unpleasant somatic symptoms would be produced. The first subsidiary hypothesis in Fast and Fisher's (1971) study was suggested by this differential: They anticipated that the higher a person's acquiescence level, the greater would be his or her anxiety when reacting to epinephrine as compared to a placebo. The greater number of somatic effects that epinephrine would presumably produce would make it more disturbing to the highly acquiescent, and the investigators expected that acquiescence would correlate positively with the report of more subjective effects resulting from epinephrine rather than from placebo. A second subsidiary hypothesis Fast and Fisher proposed was that the greater a person's acquiescence, the more likely he or she was to report epinephrine and placebo effects as occurring in interior rather than in exterior regions of the body. This idea evolved from Fisher's (1970) finding that "when persons report the sites of their body sensations over a period of time, the predominance of interior over exterior sensations correlates positively with acquiescence" (Fast and Fisher 1971, p. 67). Fisher (1970b) had pointed out that self-steering or autonomous attitudes are accompanied by an accentuated awareness of the boundary regions of the body and a minimized awareness of the body interior. An acquiescent orientation, which is presumably the opposite of an autonomous one, should therefore be typified by more awareness of interior rather than exterior body regions. The third subsidiary hypothesis was that the greater a person's acquiescence, the greater the subjective effects he or she would experience on a placebo. This prediction was based on Fisher and Fisher's (1964) report that the number of symptoms stimulated by a placebo correlates with acquiescence.

In the first experimental session, thirty college students (fifteen males and fifteen females, mean ages 22.6 for the males and 22.1 for the females) who had been recruited for a small fee, were briefly medically screened in an interview (in case of contraindications for epinephrine). Then the following were administered in this order: Measure of Body Prominence; Body Focus Questionnaire; placebo (saline solution—0.9 percent sodium chloride and 0.9 percent benzyl alcohol) followed by spontaneous reports of effects; body effect rankings and ratings of anxiety level (which were likewise repeated for the remainder of the placebo and epinephrine conditions); self-administered Holtzman Ink Blots (first twenty-five blots of Form B); epinephrine injection (0.01 mg/kg, with no attempt to keep the experimenter blind—the differential responses to epinephrine and the placebo were so obvious that the experimenter had no difficulty in distinguishing them); and the Body Distortion Questionnaire. In the second session, two days later, the following were administered in this order: Measure of Body Prominence; Bass Acquiescence Scale; epinephrine (0.001 mg/kg); self-administered Holtzman Ink Blots (first twenty-five blots from Form A); and the placebo (with suggestion of gastrointestinal symptoms).

The results indicated that the average of the two placebo conditions was greater in males than in females at about the 0.20 level ($t = 1.6$). Epinephrine conditions aroused more anxiety and elicited more reports of body effects than did placebo conditions. The combined epinephrine subjective effects exceeded the combined placebo subjective effects in both males and females, and the combined epinephrine anxiety levels exceeded the combined placebo anxiety levels in both males and females. No consistent differences emerged between the combined epinephrine and combined placebo scores, with reference to the degree to which exterior (i.e., muscle and skin), as compared to interior (i.e., stomach and heart) sites were designated as the principal foci at which the effects were experienced. When the mean ranking of the effects on various body areas of combined epinephrine or combined placebo was examined, neither males nor females showed really noteworthy differences between epinephrine and placebo ranks. Two of the hypotheses pertaining to acquiescence were not supported. The number of subjective effects produced by placebo was not related to acquiescence. Interior versus exterior body localization of effects were also not related to acquiescence. The hypothesis that the greater a person's acquiescence, the more anxiety he or she would experience during epinephrine as compared to placebo was verified.

This reaffirmation of the findings of McNair et al. (1968) gives us even more assurance that acquiescence is a mediating variable in predicting placebo versus actual drug effects. Interestingly, such similar findings were obtained from a few studies using nonpatients and another using patients. Perhaps an aspect of personality that is not situation specific and that is more a trait than a state variable has finally been found to relate very significantly to placebo responsivity. We have already noted that McNair et al. (1968) said that perhaps the adverse response of acquiescers to the drug may be reflective of a combination of thoughtless, unreliable, and invalid test taking and verbal reporting; "another possibility is that acquiescers respond with exaggerated, diffuse and, hence, nondiscriminating concern to whatever somatic cues are produced by the drug" (p. 71). The latter findings (i.e., "another possibility . . . whatever somatic cues are produced by the drug") seem to have been confirmed by Fast and Fisher (1971). Also, some relationship to the comments of McNair et al. given above may be seen in the findings of Rickels and Downing (1965) who reported a study in which they clearly showed that patients above the median on a brief multiple-choice vocabulary test discriminated between an effective tranquilizer, an ineffective tranquilizer, and a placebo. The percentage of patients improving on the effective drug was high, whereas it was low with the other two treatments. Patients characterized as "low verbal" not only did not discriminate among medications, but 65 to 80 percent of them improved on each medication. Good discrimination with marked improvement was found only on the effective drug for "high verbal" patients. These results are similar to the interaction pattern found by McNair et al. (1968) after one week.

Hypnosis. What effect does hypnotizability have on placebo responsiveness? Kissel and Barrucand (1967), working on the supposition that hypnosis would facilitate conditionability and that the placebo effect could be conceptualized within the classical conditioning paradigm, designed an experiment to show that during hypnosis there is an enhancement of suggestibility and placebo responsivity as well as conditionability. Observations (but no data) on six subjects were presented. All were undergoing placebo therapy. One patient had been clinically diagnosed as diabetes insipidus (a condition characterized by extreme ingestion of water, extreme urination, and no elevation of sugar in the urine), but presented some of the symptoms of diabetes mellitus, which were thought to be psychosomatic. Another was hospitalized for chronic severe arterial hypertension; the third had residual aches following a rib fracture; the fourth had severe asthma; the fifth was an alcoholic who refused psychiatric treatment but still wished to be cured; and the sixth had been hospitalized for hysterical hemiplegia and mutism.

While under hypnosis, subjects were first given the UCS (effective medication), with suggestion of positive results, and then a placebo (seen by the investigators as the CS), with suggestion of identical positive results. No data were presented, and no quantitative comparisons were made between the placebo response with and without hypnosis, ease of conditionability with and without hypnosis, or even base levels of the variables involved. Kissel and Barrucand (1967) nonetheless made the statement that during hypnosis "there is an increase in suggestibility, placebo responsiveness and conditionability; the three factors are intimately connected" (p. 582, my translation). These claims cannot be made given this design and in the absence of data.

Glass and Barber (1961) carried out a series of experiments to test the hypothesis that a placebo administered as a "hypnosis-producing drug" was as effective as a formal trance-induction procedure in enhancing "suggestibility." Testing the hypothesis, these researchers found that with one exception, subjects attained higher scores in the placebo session than they had obtained in a previous control session. In the placebo session, subjects obtained scores as high as those they had obtained in the trance-induction session. The hypothesis was thus confirmed, but the authors, themselves wary of outright acceptance of these findings, noted that additional experiments were in progress "to determine the validity of the hypothesis under other orders of treatment presentation and under random assignment of treatments to independent groups" (Glass and Barber 1961, p. 540).

In another experiment on placebos, suggestibility, and hypnosis, Evans (1969) found that there were no systematic correlations between placebo response and reported measures of suggestibility. Placebo measures also failed to discriminate between two groups selected from the extreme ranges of susceptibility or unsusceptibility to hypnosis. The relationships, therefore, that we might expect to find between the three phenomena when all are studied simultaneously have not emerged. Perhaps the lack of demonstration of such relationships can be attributed to the dearth of experiments in this area, or to the spuriousness of the hypothesized relationships. We will not know the answers until we find out more about all three individually and until the personality variables that they have in common have been investigated further.

Summary of the Literature on the Personality of the Placebo Reactor and Some Comments and Conclusions

Despite the fact that a number of criticisms can be made of the studies in the area, the revelation of the placebo reactor's personality is not as dismal an undertaking as such criticisms might at first suggest. We have noticed a heterogeneity of subjects, complaints, and testing instruments that makes comparison of the studies difficult. The use of nonpatient subjects appreciably reduces the evological validity of many of the studies. When no pretreatment baselines of important variables are obtained, true changes following placebo administration are difficult to measure. Sometimes double-blind procedures were not followed; specification of the criteria whereby subjects were designated reactors, nonreactors, or nocebo reactors was absent or poor; n was sometimes too small for meaningful statistical analysis of the data; and evaluation tools were sometimes not validated. Even with these criticisms in mind, does a summarization of the research findings allow a picture of the placebo responder to emerge? A pooled tabulation of the research findings for both patients and nonpatients would, particularly in the light of constant criticisms of the latter, be rather meaningless, so let us look at each group separately.

A summary of the literature on the personality of *nonpatient placebo reactors* does not yield a consistent or clear personality picture. Such people have been characterized as having good social adjustment, being outgoing and enthusiastic, and having verbally and socially skilled behavior (Muller 1965). But they have also been found to have loose and vague thinking that is poorly communicated (Linton and Langs 1962). Another study (Abramson et al. 1955) found them to have better verbal performance than nonreactors. Placebo reactors have been found to be more extroverted than nonreactors (Gartner 1953, cited in Honigfeld 1964a) but other, better studies have shown them to be more introverted (Knowles and Lucas 1960; Guy 1967). Placebo reactors are less socially dominant than nonreactors (Joyce 1959; Sharp 1965). They are more passive (Linton and Langs 1962), have low self-confidence (Joyce 1959), and low self-sufficiency (Sharp 1965). They are ideationally oriented (Abramson et al. 1955) and field dependent (Shapiro et al. 1968). They are highly anxious (Sharp 1965) or moderately so (Thorn 1962; McGlashan et al. 1969—see the section on placebos and analgesia) and react with greater anxiety to epinephrine as compared to placebo (Fast and Fisher 1971). They are more neurotic than nonreactors (Knowles and Lucas 1960; Guy 1967). They are religious (Knowles and Lucas 1960; Gelfand et al. 1965; Sharp 1965), have high social desirability scores (Gelfand et al. 1965), and are highly acquiescent (Fisher and Fisher 1963; Pichot and Perse 1968; Fisher and Fisher 1964; Fast and Fisher 1971). They are suggestible (Knowles and Lucas 1960; Linton and Langs 1962) and poorly defended and have weak affect (Linton and Langs 1962).

Nonpatient nonreactors have deviant social adjustment and are less acquiescent than reactors but more acquiescent than nocebo reactors (Pichot and Perse 1968). *Weak reactors* are primarily action oriented in their adaptive efforts (Abramson et al. 1955), have much self-doubt, maintain high standards of achievement, and have high goal striving (Linton and Langs 1962). Weak reactors are more stereotyped in their thinking than high reactors (Abramson et al. 1955) and are good tempered, socially perceptive persons who use intellectualization as a defense (Linton and Langs 1962). Their affect expression is well modulated and flexible (Linton and Langs 1962). *Nonpatient nocebo reactors* are field dependent and have more inner fantasy than placebo reactors (Shapiro et al. 1968) and are less acquiescent than both reactors and nonreactors.

This picture of nonpatient placebo responders, nonresponders, and nocebo responders is certainly a contradictory one; the currently fashionable view (e.g., Shapiro 1971a) would seem to suggest that this is the case for all studies on the personality of the placebo reactor. However, in summarizing the findings of ecologically valid studies using patients as subjects, I would like to suggest otherwise.

In *studies using patients as subjects*, placebo reactors have been found to be anxious (Lasagna et al. 1954), self-centered, emotionally labile, field dependent, and have great instinctual needs (Lasagna et al. 1954). They are religious (Lasagna et al. 1954; Duke 1964). They have low verbal intelligence (Rickels 1968), with poor discrimination among medications (Rickels and Downing 1965) perhaps being reflective of this characteristic. Their pain tolerance is better than that of nonreactors (Lasagna et al. 1954). They are dependent people who have more somatic symptoms under stress and often make use of self-prescribed medications (Lasagna et al. 1954). They are moderately to highly suggestible (Steinbook et al. 1965; Duke 1964) and highly acquiescent (McNair et al. 1968). Patients who are *nonreactors* are more rigid and emotionally controlled than reactors (Lasagna et al. 1954). This picture does not seem contradictory. A confusing or contradictory picture is more likely to emerge if, first, the personality characteristics of patients and nonpatients are pooled and, second, if nonreactors are confused with nocebo reactors. This might be what Shapiro (1971b) did before he wrote that "the attempt to relate placebo effects to the patient's personality has failed ... it is possible that no definitive traits exist" (p. 455). In a similar vein, Gallimore and Turner (1977) said that "... research to date does not support the concept of 'placebo reactor' as a unitary personality type of cluster of personality traits" (p. 51). Granted, the number of studies just cited, using patients, is relatively small, but there is some consistency between these studies, which could well serve the important heuristic function necessary in this area before it can be dismissed.

Our overall picture of the placebo reactors is that they are people who depend upon, and trust in, other people's ability to help them. In view of their religiousness, the belief that others can help them does not extend only to mortals (cf. what Zweig [1931] said about the intervention of others in situations of distress). They can react to cognitive suggestions with marked, subjectively perceivable psychological and physiological changes, and if this sounds surprising, one need only consult, for example, Schachter's work on the interaction of cognitive and physiological determinants of emotional state (Schachter 1964) or, for even more dramatic and extreme examples, Richter (1957) on voodoo death and death by suggestion. The placebo reactors place much reliance on others to be the agents in their therapeutic change. They are anxious, field dependent, talkative, and emotionally labile. They cannot get along well without other people, even though at times they allow themselves to be dominated by others, especially authority figures (like physicians). The research on acquiescence has been so impressive that further research on the role of this characteristic in the placebo responder would undoubtedly yield very fruitful results. Such research, and in fact any research on the placebo effect, should not be conducted with nonpatients. Laboratory experiments are not clinical situations, and as Shapiro (1971b) wrote, "potent psychological factors in therapy are minimized or absent in the experiment" (p. 444). An experimenter is not a therapist, a subject is not a patient, and a laboratory is not a clinic.

Fisher (1967) wrote that "to conclude that placebo reactors do not exist is, to me, as patently absurd as believing that placebo behavior is so constant that one can ultimately predict the outcome in the given situation solely on the basis of personality measurement" (p. 513). If we could plan a series of experiments using patients in clearly specified situations and using an agreed-upon battery of personality-testing instruments so that results would be comparable, we might not be uncautious to assert that by systematically investigating personality and situational interactions in this way, we would progress a great deal further in defining the placebo reactor. Let us see who this personality type is: a person with a collection of traits rather than merely state attributes and a predisposition to respond to placebos. I have in mind here a diathesis-stress kind of model. Instead of talking about polarities—that is, only personality variables at one end and only situational variables at the other—we could achieve a synthesis (interaction between personality and situation) in a less extreme way.

Sarason and Smith (1971), in discussing situational versus dispositional variables in their chapter on personality in the 1971 *Annual Review of Psychology*, made some important points of great relevance to my argument. They discussed how certain personality psychologists have recently emphasized an environmental contingency and situational approach, which has also meant ignoring, deemphasizing the contribution of, or dismissing, dispositional variables. As important as stimulus factors might be, Sarason and Smith questioned the scientific wisdom of relegating personality factors to the "error term." The fallaciousness of ignoring personality variables can be seen in every study in which significant interactions emerge between personality and situational variables. They do not argue that individual difference variables are more important than environmental variables, but to dismiss the former just because they are hard to measure or to incorporate into research designs

... serves to vitiate the avowed goals of understanding human behavior. Certainly the restriction of scientific endeavors simply to the study of functional relationships between environmental variables and behavior seems at first glance to be consistent with the physical science paradigm after which many psychologists strive to model their science. But is it really? Our connection in this regard has been expressed well by Eysenck (1967, p. 5): "No physicist would dream of assessing the electrical conductivity, or the magnetic properties or the heat-resisting qualities of matter, of 'stuff in general'. . . . Much energy was spent on the construction of Mendeleev's tables of the elements precisely because one element does not behave like another. Some conduct electricity, others do not, or do so only poorly; we do not throw all these differences into some gigantic error term, and deal only with the average of all substances. But this is what experimental psychologists do, in the cause of imitating physics! It may be said that the root of many of the difficulties and disappointments found in psychological research, as well as well-known difficulties in duplicating results from one study to another, may lie in this neglect of individual differences" [Sarason and Smith 1971, pp. 393-94].

With this perspective on the role of personality in the placebo effect, we are now ready to turn to a consideration of the latter part of the personality x situational interaction.

7

Situational Analyses of the Placebo Effect

We have examined the nature of the placebo itself, a number of conditions in which placebos have been studied, and the personality of the person taking the placebo. But we have yet to look at the milieu in which these actions occur. Several studies have been carried out to examine the way in which various situational factors, viewed as identifiable and sometimes controllable and manipulable independent variables, might be related to the placebo effect. The placebo effect was defined at the beginning of this book as "that portion of the behavioral change that can be attributed to any therapeutic procedure that is without specific activity for the condition to be treated, as contrasted to the behavioral change due to mere passage of time, repeated testing, or other 'spontaneous' influences occurring while on placebo." A definition of the placebo effect provided by Whitehorn (1958; cited in Goldstein 1962, p. 98) places emphasis on expectational and relationship considerations, with the placebo effect being seen as ". . . all those psychological and psychophysiological benefits or determinants which quite directly involve the patient's expectations that depend directly upon the diminution or augmentation of the patient's apprehension by the symbolism of the medication or the symbolic implications of the physician's behavior and attitudes." The studies and concepts that we shall examine in this chapter deal with such behavior and attitudes: demand characteristics, instructions, instructional sets and expectancy, and various aspects of the therapist-patient relationship. Parts of several studies we shall encounter here have been considered in preceding chapters of this book.

Demand Characteristics, Instructions, Instructional Sets, and Expectancy

According to Orne (1962), a subject in a psychological experiment is generally assumed, at least implicitly, to be a passive responder to stimuli. Stimuli are rigorously defined in terms of what is done to the subject, but what does the human subject *do* in the laboratory? Both subject and experimenter have well-understood roles and role expectations. The subject is usually remarkably compliant in the relationship and wishes to be a "good subject." In order to validate the experimental hypothesis, the totality of cues that convey an experimental hypothesis to the subject become significant determiners of his or her behavior. The sum total of such cues are known as the demand characteristics of the experimental situation.

A subject's behavior in any experimental situation will be determined by two sets of variables: first, the traditionally defined experimental variables and, second, the perceived demand characteristics of the experimental situation. The extent to which the subject's behavior is related to demand characteristics, rather than to the experimental variables, will in large measure determine both the extent to which the experiment can be replicated with minor modification (i.e., modified demand characteristics) and the extent to which generalizations about the effect of experimental variables in nonexperimental contexts (i.e., the problem of ecological validity) can be drawn. An important aspect to remember here is that demand characteristics result from the subject's *active* attempt to respond appropriately to the totality of the experimental situation. Imagining that an experiment could be created without demand characteristics is futile (just as is hoping that patients who are conscious will not respond to even an active medication without at least some placebo effect). Demand characteristics can be determined in several ways, for example, by systematic study of each individual subject's perception of the experimental hypothesis, through pre- or postexperimental inquiry, or by attempting to hold the demand characteristics constant and eliminate the experimental variable through the use of simulating subjects (as is often done in studies of hypnosis). The same type of technique can be utilized in other types of studies; for example, in contrast to the placebo control in a drug study, some subjects can be instructed not to take the medication at all but to act as if they had. What must be emphasized here is that this type of control is different from the placebo control because it represents an approximation. It confronts the simulating subject with a problem-solving situation and suggests how much of the total effect can be accounted for by demand characteristics. It assumes, not necessarily correctly, that the experimental group had taken full advantage of demand characteristics.

Quite conceivably, what Orne said about demand characteristics could be true of any therapeutic intervention too: Doctor and patient each have well-understood roles and role exepctations. However, doctor-patient and experimenter-subject expectations might be quite different, so that one is struck by the bearing of Orne's views on the ecological validity of nonpatient placebo experiments. When conducting experiments on placebos using patients as subjects (as opposed to "mere" treatment in which no *experimental* procedure per se is involved), the demand characteristics might be compounded to a considerable extent, since the demand characteristics of the experiment itself, as well as those involved anyway in the act of taking medicine, are both operative in such a case. The problem of demand characteristics would therefore appear to have considerable bearing on the placebo effect.

A search of the literature to date reveals only one study that specifically examines the role of demand characteristics in the placebo effect. Bank (1969) hypothesized the placebo effect to be a function of the demand characteristics of the situation, coupled with the patient's tendency to be socially desirable.

The subjects were hospitalized patients suffering from respiratory diseases (mainly tuberculosis). All patients completed the Marlowe Crowne Scale of Social Desirability; three of the Psychiatric Outpatient Mood Scales (vigor, fatigue, depression) were administered for three successive days, and on the fourth day, the experimenter, playing the role of a doctor, gave each patient a placebo capsule. The experimenter expressed a highly confident expectation of improvement with half of the subjects, and pessimism and a suggestion of no improvement with the other half. Half the patients received a placebo with inert dye added to change urine color; the other half received an ordinary lactose placebo. All of these placebos were administered for the following three days by a nurse (whether or not this phase was double-blind was not stated). The Mood Scale measurements were repeated during this time. A postexperimental interview was conducted to obtain patients' global ratings on how the placebo had affected them in general, together with patients' perceptions of the experimenter's attitudes about the placebo (as a check on the validity of the experimental manipulation). An attempt to assess the effect of the social milieu upon the placebo effect was made by questioning each patient about what he or she had heard from other persons about the "medication."

A summary of the principal findings showed that the sample as a whole, regardless of treatment, demonstrated a mild, overall placebo effect. Subjects tended to improve, regardless of whether the "doctor" expressed a confident or pessimistic attitude and regardless of whether the patient was confronted with bogus evidence of physiological change (urine cues). Social desirability was predictive of placebo response when such response involved denying unpleasant symptoms. Subjects who were high scorers on social desirability were not stronger placebo responders when such response involved making benevolent statements about placebo therapy. Bank (1969) therefore concluded that his investigation provided rather little support for the hypothesis that the placebo effect was a function of the demand characteristics of this particular placebo group situation.

The placebo effect is the behavioral consequence that results from the demand characteristics (Orne 1962) that are both perceived and responded to, so that in any given context there are many demand characteristics inherent in the situation and the subject responds only to those aspects of the demand characteristics that are perceived. Not all aspects of the demand characteristics that are perceived at some level by the subject will have a behavioral consequence. In Bank's (1969) experiment, subjects were asked in the postexperimental interview about their perceptions of the experimenter's *attitudes about the placebo* as a check on the validity of the experimental manipulation. They were not asked about *their* perceptions of the experimental manipulation, nor about their perceptions of the bogus evidence of physiological change. We cannot assert that no demand characteristics were present just because Bank failed to check on the patients' perceptions of the demand characteristics.

Nonetheless the experiment may have provided rather little support for the placebo effect's being due, in part, to demand characteristics because the subjects did not perceive any. Clearly, the extent to which demand characteristics are involved in the placebo effect warrants further and better study.

When subjects are actually told that a pill will, for example, have stimulating effects, we are dealing with a situation rather less subtle than demand characteristics. The role expectations and set can have in determining responses is well known in psychology, and, as Goldstein (1962) wrote, "[a]n individual's expectations, regarding a wide variety of human behaviors, have been demonstrated to be a potent influence shaping the form these behaviors actually take" (p. 1). The placebo effect, as we shall now see, can be a function of the deliberate manipulation of the subject's motives and expectations.

Earlier, we encountered the experiment by Guy (1967) who manipulated "environmental set" by administering Thorazine in an unfamiliar capsule with the instructional set that it was a less-potent drug than Thorazine. This study can be criticized here because of its low ecological validity, and one cannot help having the impression that particularly when attempting situational analyses, the use of nonpatient subjects is a poor analogue to the placebo-giving situation with patients. Despite this criticism, a very brief statement of Guy's results as related to this section will be given here. There were significant differences shown on both the behavioral and autonomic levels when the response to Thorazine was compared to that of the capsule—that is, the placebo. The frequencies of symptoms reported under these two conditions did not differ significantly, but the kinds of symptoms reported were different. All differences were in the direction that was predicted by the instructions minimizing the potency of the capsule. In addition, the response curve on the dynamometer task obtained by subjects who received the capsule was significantly different from that of the subjects who received the Thorazine tablet.

Experimental investigations of placebo effects on psychomotor ability were conducted by Horvath (1965). The placebo experiments were conducted on subjects appearing for their driving tests. Reactions in the optico- and acousticomotor areas were measured after the administration of placebo pills, which subjects were told were either stimulants or tranquilizers. The results showed that "the suggestive effect of placebo loading has normalized the equilibrium of stimulating-inhibiting processes within the central processes of absorbing and assimilating stimuli" (Horvath 1965, p. 105). The results also showed that the placebo effect depended on the subject's view of the drug as a stimulant or tranquilizer. Another finding was that the placebo influenced psychomotor performance of the subjects to no smaller degree than energizer or tranquilizer drugs.

Brodeur (1965) investigated the effects of placebos with stimulant suggestion and placebos with tranquilizer suggestion on forty-five senior pharmacy students who were performing their normal duties in dispensing laboratory class.

Despite the fact that this experiment was actually conducted in a pharmacy laboratory, the milieu was one to which the subjects were accustomed, and ingestion of drugs under these circumstances is not entirely unusual. Fifteen subjects were told that they had taken an amphetamine-like stimulant, fifteen that they had taken a meprobamate-like tranquilizer, and fifteen that they were controls and had taken placebo. All subjects, in actuality, took tablets filled with cornstarch. Statements suggesting the usual effects of the drugs were read to the subjects while they were in their dispensing laboratory class. The results of one pre- and two postingestion checklist scores indicated a definite trend toward placebo effects in the expected directions. Analysis of covariance showed that the differences between the groups were not significant. However, the direction of the curves on checklist scores for the stimulant and tranquilizer groups did indicate that "a possible placebo effect, due to suggestion, had taken place" (Brodeur 1965, p. 447). Pulse rates were also found to be significantly affected in the expected directions for the "drug" groups. The introspective reports at the end of the experiment indicated that 60 percent of the subjects felt the drug effect they were told to expect, with the greatest number of effects being reported by the stimulant group. Placebo effects were felt by 73.3 percent of subjects in the "stimulant" group and 46.7 in the "tranquilizer" group. No percentages were reported for the introspective reports in the control group. The pressures of the situation in which the study was carried out (i.e., the usual rushed atmosphere of a laboratory class) might, according to the author, have been the reason for the largest placebo effect in the "stimulant" group. "The results of this study clearly indicate that suggestion, in the form of placebos and instructions, can play a role in effecting a feeling of stimulation or tranquilization in healthy subjects" (Brodeur 1965, p. 449). Even though the author mentions that the wording of the instructions might have accounted for a large part of the effects, the mere use of the word "suggestion" without explaining exactly what is meant is, as we have already seen, a very unsatisfactory attempt at explaining why placebo effects occur.

Thomas and Hull (1971) measured two-point thresholds on the forearms of fourteen volunteer subjects from an introductory psychology course. In the simulated drug threshold part of the experiment, some xylocaine was placed on the tongue of each subject, thereby producing numbness. When vaseline, believed to be the same active anesthetic, was applied to their arms, the two-point threshold was significantly increased in nearly two-thirds of the subjects who gave affirmative reports of numbness on their arms. When the same placebo was used and subjects were informed that a control test was being conducted and that vaseline was being used instead of xylocaine, and these results were compared with those in the placebo condition, the percentage increase of mean placebo threshold over mean control threshold for each subject ranged from −10 percent to +45 percent.

Several experiments demonstrating observable physiological changes following placebo ingestion and instructions have been reported. Volunteer subjects were tested on three occasions by Sternbach (1964) after being told how their stomachs would feel following the ingestion of a "drug" (placebo). First, in the "stimulant drug" condition, they were told that soon after taking the pill a strong churning sensation would be felt in their stomachs. On the second occasion, a so-called "relaxant" drug was given, and subjects were told that it would make their stomachs feel full and heavy. The third occasion was presented to subjects as a placebo control condition with which the effects of the first two "drugs" could be compared. What the subjects actually swallowed was a gelatin capsule containing a small magnetic tracer that allowed stomach movements to be recorded. Four of the six subjects tested showed marked stomach changes exactly in line with what they had been told to expect.

Frankenhaeuser, Jaerpe, Svan, and Wrangsjoe (1963) conducted an experiment on the effects of a "depressant" and a "stimulant" placebo on various objective and subjective reactions of female subjects. Their first visit to the laboratory was made so that subjects could familiarize themselves with the experimental procedure. Two more sessions followed, on one of which each subject took two white gelatin capsules, reputedly a "sleep-producing drug," while on the other visit two pink gelatin capsules containing a "stimulant drug" were administered. Both the white and the pink capsules were placebos. Several physiological measures were taken throughout each session, and in addition each subject was asked to say whether she felt subjectively quicker or slower and more or less alert, sleepy, happy, and depressed than before she had taken the "drug." The two types of placebo clearly had opposite effects on all measures taken, with all the changes being in the predicted direction and with the alterations in subjective state being paralleled by changes on a reaction time test that was also given: On the "stimulant" the subjects showed a faster response pattern, with a rise in heart rate and blood pressure, while the opposite effects occurred after subjects took the "depressant" placebo.

Another experiment by Frankenhaeuser and her colleagues (Frankenhaeuser, Post, Hagdahl, and Wrangsjoe 1964) showed how under certain conditions, even an active drug can produce changes quite different from those it normally produces. Reactions of subjects under three conditions were studied. Subjects in the first condition were given a placebo and told that, like a depressant-type drug, it would have typical sleep-producing effects. Both of the other conditions involved the administration of quite a potent dose (200 mg) of pentobarbital. In the first of these pentobarbital conditions, subjects were told to expect the usual depressant effects. In the other pentobarbital condition, subjects were told that the drug might or might not have any effect at all. Analysis of various measurements taken on the subjects on the three occasions (e.g., reaction time, ratings of various subjective feelings) revealed that irrespective of the treatment, the substance given had a consistently significant effect only when it was combined with the appropriate suggestions beforehand. Neutral instructions resulted in a rather weak effect.

What happens when subjects are told they will be receiving a drug and the brand name of a familiar drug is given? Morris and O'Neal (1974) devised a test for differing predictions about the relationship of drug name familiarity and the placebo effect. Four different drug names were used: Two had the names of commonly known drugs, and two had fictitious names. All were actually placebos. Subjects were sixty-four male students who volunteered to participate in this "drug study" for a chance to win a lottery prize. They were told that the purpose of the research was to assess the effects of certain drugs on psychomotor skills and recall. The task was a pursuit rotor one. There were several variables in this study. Analysis of the one we are interested in here, the familiarity variable, did not reveal any significant effects for drug familiarity. As Morris and O'Neal (1974) stated, "Perhaps familiarity with the name of a drug is not in itself a strong enough variable, and actual experience with the drug may be necessary for familiarity to affect [the conditioning or attribution process]" (p. 281). We shall see more about conditioning and attribution in the chapter on theoretical explanations of the placebo effect. For the moment, however, we see that drug name familiarity did not seem to be of importance in contributing to a placebo effect in *healthy* subjects. Whether this finding would be the same for patients still needs to be examined. Such experiments would be easy to design. Positive results might even increase the frequency with which we would be bombarded with advertising that tries to impress one drug name or another on us!

What happens when no specific instructions are actually given and patients are told that they are receiving placebos? We have seen that sometimes they react as one would expect them to under these circumstances—i.e., no effect—as in the study by Thomas and Hull (1971). A whole study was designed by Park and Covi (1965) to test this question. Fifteen newly admitted neurotics were administered placebos in an outpatient setting. Each patient was seen twice: During the first visit they were evaluated and placebos were prescribed, and the second visit, which took place one week later, consisted of two separate interviews aimed at assessing change and making further disposition. Two psychiatrists participated, one of whom served as therapist for eight patients and the other, for seven. Each interview was observed through a one-way screen by one of the psychiatrists who also tape recorded the session and interviewed the patient at the end of the second session.

When the patients were given the placebos, they were told that they were getting "sugar pills," which had helped many other patients and which they were to take t.i.d. at mealtimes. They were asked to discontinue taking any other psychoactive drug they might have been taking at the time. The third visit consisted of a brief interview focused on present symptoms and on changes that had occurred since the the first visit. The other psychiatrist then further explored with the patient the changes noticed in the patient's feelings and opinions about the treating doctor and the treatment received and the patient's desires concerning future treatment. Four improvement measures were used:

overall change, symptom checklist, target symptoms, and pathology. Fourteen of the fifteen patients returned for the second visit.

The results showed that on the symptom checklist, thirteen of the fourteen patients improved; on the target symptoms, all fourteen improved; and on the pathology ratings, twelve patients improved, one was rated as unchanged, and one was worse. On the average patient overall change score, thirteen improved and one reported no change, and on the doctor overall change ratings, all patients improved. Eleven patients improved on all measures, and there were no significant differences in improvement scores of patients seen by one or the other doctor. *The interviews showed that even though they had been told they were receiving placebos, improvement occurred in the eight patients believing this information.* The six patients who believed that they had received an active drug even though they had been told that they were to receive placebos also improved, and in fact there were no significant differences between the two groups. Improvement was not related to belief that the pills were or were not placebos, but did appear to be related to certainty of belief regarding the nature of the pills: The three patients who definitely believed that they had received placebos, as well as the two who were absolutely certain that they had received active drugs, all improved more than the other nine. The five patients dealing with the treatment situation in a relatively stereotyped way—patterned on previous doctor and medication experiences—tended to believe that they were helped chiefly by an active drug, and the other nine patients tended to believe that they were helped by the placebo, by themselves, or by the doctor. Seemingly, even if some neurotic outpatients know that they are receiving inert pills, they will still take them and will improve. At least five of the patients even desired to continue the placebo treatment, and two felt in no need of further treatment. Furthermore, unawareness of the inert nature of the placebo is not an indispensable condition for improvement. The above study was not without its methodological problems. For example, the sample size was small enough to present the chance that a large percentage of the persons who were included would have improved markedly under any treatment.

We have seen that instructions can markedly influence the placebo effect, not only in terms of the psychological effects reported, but also in observable physiological changes that occur. Schachter (1964) has shown that given a state of physiological arousal for which a person has no explanation, he or she will label this state in terms of the cognitions available, and given a state of physiological arousal for which the person has a completely satisfactory explanation, this state will not be labeled in terms of the alternative cognitions available. Let us look at what might happen when a placebo is administered. Theoretically, if we assume that there is no sympathetic activation when a placebo is ingested, the state we are measuring might have an extremely low value: Schachter's theory would predict that since emotional state is a joint function of a state of physiological arousal and of the appropriateness of a cognition, we are, in effect, assuming a multiplicative function so that if either component is at zero, emotional level is at zero. However, not only do we have experimental evidence that placebos do produce some physiological arousal (and in fact any placebo-giving situation in which there is no arousal whatsoever is virtually impossible to imagine), but we can also see that the necessary cognitive labels were readily supplied by the experimenters in the form of the instructions given to the subjects in the studies we have examined thus far in this chapter. Therefore, given a state of physiological arousal for which subjects have a satisfactory explanation, they will often experience what they have been told they will experience. Indeed, a study by Weiner and Valins (unpublished; results cited in Weiner 1971) found that if subjects in a fearful situation were informed that a placebo caused the psychological symptoms of arousal, they would infer that the placebo was also the cause of the physiological symptoms of arousal.

Examining what happens when subjects misattribute the physiological or psychological symptoms separately or in combination is of interest here. Weiner (1971) conducted a study in which half of the subjects were first given a placebo and then informed that the research involved exposing them to a series of rather painful electric shocks (placebo-arousal), with the sequence reversed (arousal-placebo) for the other half of the subjects. Weiner investigated, first, the importance of the contiguity between the onset of arousal and the administration of a placebo upon fear reduction, and second, the nature of the symptoms that were attributed to the placebo. The total symptom attribution group was informed that the pill produced both the physiological and psychological side effects of fear. The physiological symptom attribution group and the psychological symptom attribution group were informed that the pill caused only physiological or only psychological arousal, respectively. The subjects were told that the physiological symptoms would be palpitations, palm perspiration, and genreal visceral upset, and the psychological symptoms would be "nervous, tense, and jumpy." The fourth group was informed that the pill would cause symptoms that were actually totally irrelevant (although subjects were not aware of this total irrelevance) to arousal resulting from fear of shock—that is, stuffiness of the auditory and nasal passages and itchiness over parts of the body.

The results indicated that the placebo-arousal *sequence* had no effect upon misattribution of symptoms nor upon fear reduction. However, the two groups that had been told that the placebo would cause physiological arousal—total-symptom attribution and physiological-symptom attribution—attributed significantly less arousal to the electric shock than did the psychological symptom attribution and irrelevant symptom attribution groups. Similar scores were obtained for the attribution of psychological arousal. Weiner (1971) wrote that "[a]ccording to the attribution data, only the total-symptom attribution group, since they misattributed both physiological and psychological arousal, should have shown evidence of fear reduction" (p. 1218). What Weiner called "misattribution" in this experiment was, however, really the placebo effect: Subjects were told that the *placebo* would produce various physiological and/or psychological symptoms, and so there was some confounding here. That these are also the symptoms that can be produced when people anticipate electric shock does not mean that they were of necessity *mis*attributed to the placebo. What Weiner actually obtained here can possibly be viewed as more data in support of a Schachter-like interpretation of the placebo effect where the subjects experience symptoms, both physiological and psychological, that they had been told to expect (i.e., a cognition is readily available).

At the beginning of this chapter, we extended our definition of the placebo effect to include Whitehorn's (1958) emphasis on expectational and relationship considerations. We have looked at the expectational considerations, and in the next section of this chapter, we shall examine what is involved in the relationship considerations of the expanded definition. We shall examine therapeutic milieu, the therapist-patient relationship, and therapist characteristics.

Therapeutic Milieu: The Therapist-Patient Relationship and the Personality of the Therapist

What do we know about the way in which patients react to placebos in particular types of therapeutic situations, and what is the relationship between various therapist characteristics and the way in which these therapists' patients react to placebos (or active drugs, for that matter)? In the Introduction to this book, we noted that Ellenberger (1970) had written that "the primitive healer exerts his action primarily through his personality, whereas the scientific therapist applies scientific techniques in an impersonal way. The primitive healer is primarily a psychosomatician, treating many physical diseases by psychological techniques, but in scientific therapy there is a dichotomy between physical and psychic therapy" (p. 47). Let us examine the evidence in an attempt to find answers to the questions posed·at the beginning of this paragraph and at the same time discover that Ellenberger's distinctions do not really hold.

We have already examined and criticized very briefly the study by Lowinger and Dobie (1969) in which the effectiveness of placebos in outpatients visiting a drug clinic was studied. Lowinger and Dobie's study as published was actually a report on a series of substudies, each of which was performed in the larger context of drug evaluations and with each having a placebo control. The percentage of schizophrenic patients ranged from 30 percent to 50 percent, and the remainder of the subjects were divided between those with personality disorders and psychoneurosis, depending on the particular substudy. Placebo response rates ranged from 24 percent to 76 percent in the four substudies, but unfortunately no breakdown of the placebo responsivity for each diagnostic category was given. Lowinger and Dobie found that the *milieu* in which the drugs and placebos were administered exerted considerable effects on the patients' chances for improvement. The placebo response rates in the four double-blind outpatient substudies were 24 percent, 35 percent, 74 percent, and 76 percent. The psychosocial variables responsible for these differences are of interest to us here.

A study using large doses of the active drug tends to be an impressive therapeutic endeavor, even when a physician does not know whether a patient is being given active drugs or placebos. Doctors are more enthusiastic about this type of double-blind study. They are also more alert to toxicity and convey this to the patient even in very subtle ways. Doctors who take part in double-blind studies in which they know the drugs are milder, or are used in smaller dosages, are possibly less optimistic about how patients will change therapeutically. They are also less concerned about toxicity. In addition to all these factors concerning the physician, Lowinger and Dobie (1969) also found that a study requiring frequent tests offers an extended emotional experience. Through frequent appearances at the location of treatment, the patient gains additional support and identification from the research personnel, some of whom may well be identified with the therapeutic endeavor, thereby increasing the emotional impact that results in symptom relief. We have already seen that even double-blind procedures are not immune to nonspecific effects, and Lowinger and Dobie's study was useful in that it pointed out where this immunity can break down.

Another study showing that many situational factors can influence the results of a double-blind study was reported by Constant and Dubois (1975). They showed how a whole series of relationships in a hospital can be threatened by such a study. The nurse-patient relationship, the nurse-doctor relationship, and the relationship of the doctor to the drug under study were all examined before studying the pharmacological effect of the active drug (i.e., the drug-patient relationship). Constant and Dubois showed how, in examining such relationships, an institution can actually do things to lead to improvements in the services it provides.

A number of situational variables that influence placebo effects have been documented by Shapiro (1971a): Staff attitudes, expectations, biases, conflicts, and harmony of the staff can influence placebo effects, as can subject and patient population, treatment procedure, and miscellaneous factors. For example, regarding staff attitudes, Shapiro stated that one study revealed that patients treated with placebos improved more than patients on tranquilizers; this finding was attributed to the bias of the nurses *against* psychochemotherapy and *for* habit-training psychotherapy. The nurses were observed crushing, dissolving, and tasting the tablets in order to distinguish between the placebo and the active agent! Treatment procedure may vary insofar as the type of placebo or drug, the instructions, and so forth are concerned. Important miscellaneous factors are spontaneous remission, transient everyday symptoms, new social group formation, and change of environment.

Even though the relationship between the doctor and the patient has been recognized throughout history as an important determinant of the response to treatment, a deemphasis on how the *person* of the physician (rather than his or her expert knowledge) contributes to the placebo effect and to therapeutic effects was almost a rule for scores of years. However, as Shapiro (1971a) noted, research conducted recently on the role of the physician in placebo and therapeutic effects makes us see how critical a variable the psychosociology of the physician is in therapy. In 1964, Shapiro coined the term *iatroplacebogenics* to describe the study of placebo effects produced by physicians (Shapiro 1964b). Shapiro (1971a) views *direct iatroplacebogenics* as "placebo effects produced by the direct effect of the physician's attitude to the patient, treatment and the results of treatment" (p. 605), and *attitude toward the patient* refers to the therapist's "interest, warmth, liking, sympathy, empathy, neutrality, disinterest, hostility and rejection" (p. 605). Shapiro reported one study that showed that the physician's personal interest, and not the physician's competence, was the main determinant of whether or not patients like their doctors. Goldstein (1962) found that patient-physician expectations are important in therapy: Therapists' favorable feelings to patients are related to the therapists' expectation of improvement and the patients' attraction to the therapist and thus influence the attained improvement.

According to Shapiro (1971a), *attitude toward treatment* in direct iatroplacebogenesis "such as the therapist's faith, belief, enthusiasm, conviction, commitment, optimism, interest, positive and negative expectations, skepticism, disbelief, and pessimism about treatment, has been established by research as a nonspecific factor in most therapies" (p. 606). Differentiating between the therapist's interest in the patient and treatment is difficult, but quite a few studies suggest that the therapist's interest in treatment is frequently primary and leads to a secondary interest in the patient. The sequence here is interesting: The patient's hope and optimism are mobilized by the therapist's interest in the treatment. *Attitude toward results* (Shapiro, 1971a) refers to the investigator's interests that result in data distortion caused by random observer bias. Support for the inclusion of this factor comes from, for example, Rosenthal's work on biases like observer bias and the relation of experimenter bias to the experimenter's hypotheses, expectations, motivation, prestige, and so forth. An interest in results can directly effect a nonrandom intentional or unintentional observer bias. "Data are influenced, communicated, distorted, and then used to confirm hypotheses" (Shapiro 1971a, p. 607). *Indirect placebogenesis*, according to Shapiro (1971a), refers to the fact that the physician's interest may be indirect, subtle, and paradoxical. Placebo effects may be attributable to the physician's or therapist's interest in a particular theory or method of treatment. The physician may not really be interested in the patient, but the patient may experience the physician's interest in the treatment as a personal one. "Thus, placebo effects are produced or augmented when the physician is prestigious, dedicated to his [or her] theory or therapy, especially if it is his [or her] own innovation, or if he [or she] is a recent convert; and when the therapies are elaborate, detailed, expensive, time-consuming, fashionable, esoteric, and dangerous" (Shapiro 1971a, p. 608).

Let us now look at studies on "Who makes treatment work?" One of the best early studies carried out on what amounts to "Who makes the placebo work for neurotic patients?" was published by Uhlenhuth, Canter, Neustadt, and Payson (1959), who designed a double-blind study with meprobamate, phenobarbital, and a placebo in such a way as to permit comparisons on the patients of two psychiatrists who had been previously selected to differ strikingly on certain specific criteria. The patients were psychoneurotic outpatients with anxiety symptoms and were referred to the study by part-time psychiatrists at the clinic the patients attended. The patients were screened for organic brain syndrome, alcoholism, psychosis, and severe intellectual deficit, and then assigned to two well-matched groups, A or B, with equal distribution of sex, race, age, marital status, diagnostic classification, and initial symptom checklist scores. Twenty-six patients in each group completed the study.

Each patient received either meprobamate (400 mg q.i.d.), phenobarbital (16 mg q.i.d.), or placebo q.i.d. for two weeks, with each medication being given first for a third of the patients. Each psychiatrist was chosen as representative of certain contrasting patterns on the Strong Vocational Interest Bank (but the actual data for these differences were not specified by the investigators). Dr. A was noticeably younger and less fatherly than Dr. B and did not, in contrast to Dr. B, expect that there would be differences in the effectiveness of the medications. Dr. A's manner was noncommital, Dr. B's more hopeful. Patients after treatment endorsed Dr. B as "helpful" and "dependable" significantly more often than Dr. A. Dr. A treated group A, Dr. B treated group B, and each patient saw his or her doctor at bi-weekly intervals for brief interviews directed toward completing progress report forms in order to minimize nonpharmacological therapeutic effects.

The three measures used were the patient's overall judgment (better, same, or worse), the doctor's overall judgment, and a forty-five-symptom checklist. All judgments were related to the patient's condition at the first interview, the three measures for each interview were pooled, and the patient was considered improved if at least two measures agreed in this judgment (these data did not give information about the *extent* of improvement). At the end of six weeks, 81 percent of the patients were improved. When improvement at the end of each two-week medication was analyzed, the investigators found that in the total patient population, there were no significant differences in effectiveness among the three medications. However, when the results were analyzed according to which group the patient belonged to, they found that in Dr. A's group about the same number of patients was improved after treatment with each drug and placebo, while in Dr. B's group, more patients tended to improve on meprobamate and phenobarbital than on placebo. Uhlenhuth et al. noted the striking correlation between what the doctor expected from the medication and how his group responded to them. "Dr. A expected no marked differences [between active drugs and placebo] and none appeared.... The psychiatrist's expectations may operate in at least two ways. His expectation that the drugs have like effects may raise his own and his patient's perceptual threshold for differences in effectiveness. His expectation that the drugs have different effects may lower these thresholds. [Second,] the psychiatrist who expects differences is likely to show more interest. This may produce an emotional state in the patient which heightens his responses to differences in pharmacologic effect.... Some of the investigator's expectations regarding the effectiveness of treatment may influence the results, in spite of the double-blind design" (Uhlenhuth et al. 1959, pp. 908-09). Quite clearly, Ellenberger's (1970) comment, cited at the beginning of this book, to the effect that primitive healers exert their action primarily through their personalities, whereas the scientific therapist applies scientific techniques in an impersonal way needs some rethinking in the light of these results and similar ones of other studies, which we will examine now.

We saw that the personality variables derived from the SVIB were not given in detail by Uhlenhuth et al. (1959). The results of a study in which more detailed doctor characteristics, as well as those of patients (thus fulfilling the patient x situational variables interaction about which we talked at the end of the section on the personality of the placebo reactor), by Rickels, Cattell, Weise, Gray, Yee, Mallin, and Aaronson (1966) were presented in summarized form in Rickels' (1968b) paper at the Fourth World Congress of Psychiatry, Madrid, 1966. Patients in private psychiatric practice were treated with psychotherapy and additionally received either 1600 mg per day of meprobamate or placebo, under double-blind conditions, for six weeks. Prior to the study onset, psychiatrists completed several personality tests and attitudinal scales. The evaluation of patients was conducted every two weeks. Psychiatrists scoring high on authoritarianism (California F Scale) and extroversion were defined—according to a measure derived from the SVIB by Betz (1963)—as Type A physicians. Type A physicians have been reported to achieve better results with psychiatric drugs than psychiatrists who scored lower on the two measures and who were defined as Type B physicians. Four of the five participating psychiatrists could be divided, based on the personality variables mentioned above, into two groups of two physicians each. Group I psychiatrists were predicted by Rickels, Cattell et al. (1966) to do well, and Group II psychiatrists to do poorly in drug treatment of their patients.

Drug-placebo differences in the patients in the two groups were compared, and the results demonstrated that patients in Group I improved significantly more on drug than placebo, while those in Group II responded well to placebo. The hypothesis was thus confirmed, but the differential placebo response was not understood. The two patient populations were therefore compared on demographic and predictor variables. Patients of the more authoritarian-type, more extroverted doctors (Group I psychiatrists) were "sicker, more chronically ill, more drug pretreated, older, less educated, and expressed a strong desire for therapy alone. . . . In other words, those patients represented exactly the type of patients who are expected from clinical experience to do better with a combination of psychotherapy and drugs than with psychotherapy alone. In contrast, the patients of the less authoritarian, less extroverted, type B doctors, i.e. the psychotherapy-oriented doctors (Group II psychiatrists), much more represented the *typical* psychotherapy patient. These patients were of lower initial psychopathology, more acutely ill, less drug pretreated, better educated, younger, and expected primarily only psychotherapy and not drug therapy. Such a patient usually does well on placebo" (Rickels 1968b, pp. 15-16). This study illustrates the complexity of what can happen: Psychiatrists who differed according to three personality variables treated patients who also differed in a consistent and meaningful way on several variables. Perhaps a set of patient-related nonspecific factors that affected therapy outcome occurred as a function of physician characteristics because physicians either selected these patients differentially or had attracted over the years a different patient population. Maybe a strong possibility exists that a private psychiatrist attracts a certain type of patient for therapy—that is, a patient who fits his or her own personality, attitudes, and expectations.

Two studies on the effects of doctors' and patients' attitudes and other factors in response to drugs were carried out by two hundred general practitioners in the British Isles and reported by Wheatley at the Fourth World Congress of Psychiatry, Madrid, 1966 (Wheatley 1968). The patients were anxious and depressed private patients, and the data were collected in two double-blind crossover studies conducted over a period of two months. The first study compared chlordiazepoxide and amylobarbitone in the treatment of anxiety, and the second compared imipramine and phenobarbitone in the treatment of depression. Although the study did not deal with placebos, the results will be presented here because they have impressive implications for situational studies of the placebo effect. Each doctor recorded his and each patient's attitudes toward treatment outcome, so that these attitudes varied according to the particular case. Three classifications were used for both patients and doctors—optimistic, indifferent, and pessimistic—and nine combinations were possible. In the anxiety trial, 70 doctors treated 134 patients, and in the depression trial 97 doctors treated 170 patients. Results of measures of attitudes toward treatment outcome did not differ in relation to whether the patients were anxious or depressed. Results of drug treatment showed that best results with both drugs were, as expected, obtained with the optimistic doctors, less good results with the indifferent doctors, and the worst with the pessimistic doctors. The differential response in relation to patients' attitudes was similar but the differences were not so marked. Statistical analysis of these results showed that for each individual drug, the differences between the results for optimistic, pessimistic, and indifferent doctors were all statistically significant from one another at the 5 percent level. Patients' attitudes were related as follows: On the chlordiazepoxide, the optimists showed significantly better results than indifferent and pessimistic patients (at the 5 percent level of significance), but the difference between the indifferent patients and the pessimistic ones was not significant. On amylobarbitone, there was no significant difference between optimistic patients and indifferent ones, but the difference between the results for pessimists was significantly poorer than for optimists and indifferent patients.

An interesting pattern emerged of the relationship of the effects of both doctor and patient attitudes to the improvement of anxious patients. There was a distinct pattern of highest improvement with both doctor and patient optimism, a lower level with both doctor and patient indifference, and the least improvement with both doctor and patient pessimism. In the case of depression, the results were not consistently influenced to any degree by either the doctors' or patients' attitudes. Seemingly, therefore, the effects of these attitudes, while of considerable importance in the drug treatment of anxiety, are of little importance in neurotic depression.

Wheatley also found that clinical results varied hardly at all in relation to the duration of symptoms when chlordiazepoxide was the treatment, but that results with amylobarbitone were poorer, the longer the duration of symptoms. Interestingly, the results are similar to those reported by Rickels, Lipman, and Raab (1966), whose article on previous medication, duration of illness and placebo response was examined earlier in this book. In that study, chlordiazepoxide and meprobamate were compared to placebo, and phenobarbital sodium was also compared to placebo, whereas in Wheatley's trial direct comparison was made between two active drugs. This trial therefore provided independent confirmation for the influence of this factor on drug treatment in the results of anxiety studies. Unfortunately, no placebo condition was included in Wheatley's study, which is a fascinating example of interactions between physician, patient, and drug characteristics, and a study with that amount of detail is sorely needed in the placebo literature.

As is therefore apparent, in trying to understand any treatment results in placebo therapy, both the patient variables and the physician variables must be considered. Clearly, neither one nor the other can be considered in isolation, as has been the case in the overwhelming majority of the studies we have examined. The interaction between patient, therapist, and milieu variables is so clearly what is involved in the placebo effect that experiments in which the influence of any of these is not controlled are rather shortsighted, given what we now know about these independent variables. Some of the clearest instances of the operation of all these factors are evidenced in the study of the placebo effect in psychotherapy, to which we now turn in chapter 8.

8 The Placebo Effect in Psychotherapy

In discussing the placebo effect in psychotherapy, one is faced with an interesting dilemma, because the variables of a psychological nature—the "superfluous," "nonspecific," and almost "unwanted" and "confounding" factors in drug or other physical therapies—are precisely what constitute an essential part of what psychotherapy is all about. Few writers seem to have realized this when talking about psychotherapy placebo effect. The problem arises because nothing in psychotherapy can really be called "inert" in a psychological sense, and one is faced with the question: "When is a placebo effect is psychotherapy a placebo effect?"

In order to answer this question and related ones, some general comments about psychotherapy will first be made and a definition of psychotherapy will be given. The necessary and sufficient conditions for psychotherapy will then be discussed, after which the definition of "placebo effect" will again be discussed, thereby leading to a consideration of the necessary and sufficient conditions for the placebo effect to occur. The question of how one can be assured that psychotherapeutic procedures are not merely placebogenic will then be examined. A review of some experimental studies of the placebo effect in psychotherapy will show that in many instances the so-called psychotherapy placebo is not that at all, and the necessity for distinguishing between nonspecific effects in psychotherapy and "placebo" controls in psychotherapy research will be stressed.

Psychotherapy has been called a number of things, including "the purchase of friendship" (Schofield 1964) and "the art of applying a science which does not yet exist" (cited in Meehl 1973, p. 117). The latter view is perhaps the most cynical of those that will be examined here and is one that, if accepted, leaves a rather nasty taste in the mouths of those of us who are clinicians. Anyone having even a slight acquaintance with both the broad general area of psychotherapy and the research conducted over the last twenty-five years on its effectiveness will know that this procedure has been variously praised, vilified, condemned, refuted, and admired, but nonetheless survived as an increasingly important service provided by mental health professionals. The varieties of psychotherapy are manifold and range from operant conditioning to classical Freudian psychoanalysis. Wolberg (1967) has classified the varieties of psychotherapy first in relation to the objectives they pursue and, second, the fields from which they derive their substance. Wolberg presented fairly detailed classificatory tables that will not be duplicated here (the interested reader should consult Wolberg 1967, pp. 14-15). The main types of treatment are supportive therapy, which aims at the restoration to an adaptive equilibrium through approaches like guidance and suggestive hypnosis; reeducative therapy, in which, for example, deliberate efforts are made at readjustment and goal modification through approaches like behavior therapy, client-centered therapy, and family therapy; and reconstructive therapy, which pursues such objectives as insight into unconscious conflicts with efforts to achieve extensive alterations of character structure through approaches like psychoanalysis (of all schools), existential analysis, and transactional approaches. The fields from which therapies derive their substance are biology (e.g., neuroanatomy, physiology, biochemistry, genetics) with treatment methods such as somatic therapies; psychology (e.g., learning theory, personality theory, psychoanalytic theory) with treatment methods such as behavior therapy and psychoanalysis; sociology (e.g., role theory, field theory, group dynamics) with treatment methods such as group therapy and transactional therapy; and philosophical areas involving the application, for essentially therapeutic purposes, of philosophical, religious, or other tenets of, for example, Zen Buddhism, Yoga, and existentialism. Wolberg's classification is only one of the myriad ways in which psychotherapy can be classified; such classifications are by no means fixed and definitive.

When psychotherapy is mentioned in this chapter, we shall (unless otherwise specified) be talking of the sorts of treatment mentioned above. While taking a course in positive thinking, casting a spell, or following the advice of one's favorite "lonely-hearts" columnist are not entirely unrelated to what will be discussed, the things inherent in Wolberg's (1967) definition of psychotherapy are much more closely related to and relevant to the discussion: "Psychotherapy is the treatment, by psychological means, of problems of an emotional nature in which a trained person deliberately establishes a professional relationship with the patient with the object of (1) of removing, modifying or retarding existing symptoms, (2) of mediating disturbed patterns of behavior, and (3) of promoting positive personality growth and development" (p. 3). Again, while this definition is not the only one that could be given, it is a useful one in that it emphasizes psychological means, problems of an emotional nature, trained persons, professional relationships, and symptom change.

Despite the different schools, methods, and foundations of psychotherapy, as most authors indicate, the various and diverse approaches have a great deal in common, so that even though talking about "psychotherapy" can sometimes be difficult unless one specifies which system or group of treatment systems is under consideration, once one has a definition like Wolberg's, one does at least have a guideline. Patterson (1967) has said of this problem: "To some extent the various theories or points of view represent different ways of describing or explaining the same phenomena. Differences are in part related to the use of different emphases, to different perceptions of the same events, to differences in comprehensiveness of formulation. To some extent differences may appear greater than those that actually exist. This may be due in part to the use of different terminology to the same or similar concepts. Differences may also be exaggerated by the propensity to emphasize differences rather than similarities" (p. 11).

The interesting thing that concerns us here is that when we examine the similarities between the various psychotherapeutic approaches, we find that they resemble the nonspecific elements in the research on the placebo effect that has been considered in the preceding chapters. Some of these similarities between various psychotherapeutic approaches will be mentioned here. Truax and Mitchell (1971), in an extensive literature review, found evidence suggesting that therapists or counselors who are accurately empathic, nonpossessively warm in attitude, and genuine are highly effective, with patient improvement being very strongly related to high levels of these therapeutic conditions. Low levels of accurate empathy, nonpossessive warmth, and genuineness are important factors leading to patient deterioration. These findings seem to hold with a wide variety of therapists and counselors of all theoretical orientations and types of training and with a wide variety of patients and clients. The evidence also suggests that these findings hold in a wide variety of therapeutic contexts and in both individual and group psychotherapy or counseling. The fact that the findings hold with a wide variety of therapists and counselors of all theoretical orientations suggests that accurate empathy, nonpossessiveness, and genuineness are not factors that are specific to the particular type of psychotherapy being practiced. "Attention, interest, concern, trust, faith, belief and expectation are part of what is designated as the placebo effect in the treatment of physical diseases" (Patterson, 1967); some or all of these can be considered essential in both psychotherapy and the placebo effect. Does this statement mean that psychotherapy is a placebo, and if it does not, how can we be sure that psychotherapeutic effects are more than merely placebo effects? In order to answer this question, the necessary and sufficient conditions for psychotherapeutic change will be discussed, following which the definition of "placebo effect" will again be examined, thereby leading to a consideration of the necessary and sufficient conditions for its occurrence.

Philosophers of science customarily distinguish between necessary and sufficient conditions for the occurrence of an event. A *necessary* condition for the occurrence of a specified event is "a circumstance in whose absence the event cannot occur" (Copi 1961, p. 355). A *sufficient* condition for the occurrence of an event is "a circumstance in whose presence the event must occur" (Copi 1961, pp. 355-56). What we are really talking about here is the notion of causality, and when referring to psychotherapy, the necessary conditions are easier to discuss than the sufficient ones. We may have difficulty in conceiving of events in whose presence therapeutic change *must* occur and may find the process rather easier for events in whose absence the therapeutic change cannot occur. Psychotherapeutic change is not nearly as concrete a phenomenon as is combustion, the example given by Copi to illustrate the necessary and sufficient conditions in a chemical event. The presence of oxygen is a necessary condition for combustion to occur; if combustion occurs, then oxygen must have been present. In psychotherapy, if therapeutic change occurs, can we point to the presence of x such that we can make the statement "the presence of x is a necessary condition for psychotherapeutic change to occur; if psychotherapeutic change occurs, then x must have been present"? Let us hold the answer until we repeat the same question with the sufficient conditions for psychotherapeutic change by again taking combustion as a more concrete example. The presence of oxygen is a necessary but not a sufficient condition for combustion to occur since oxygen can be present without combustion occurring. However, a temperature range exists such that for any substance, being in the presence of oxygen is a sufficient condition for the combustion of that substance. There may be several necessary conditions for combustion, and they must all be included in the sufficient condition. In psychotherapy, if therapeutic change occurs, can we then point to the presence of events x, y, and z such that we can say "the presence of x, y, z are sufficient conditions for psychotherapeutic change to occur; if psychotherapeutic change occurs, then x, y, z must have been present"?

There are a number of ways in which this question has been answered. Ellis (1959) criticized the necessary and sufficient conditions proposed by Rogers (1957) and concluded that while there are no necessary conditions, a number of sufficient conditions do exist. Unless we are talking of a specific type of psychotherapy, this position appears to be quite acceptable, especially if we use the generic "psychotherapy" to refer to all the different therapeutic results. The only common element all types have that would approach being the necessary *and* sufficient condition for psychotherapy is the relationship between two people—that is, between the patient and the therapist. The sufficient conditions would appear to be those mentioned above, for example, accurate empathy, attention, trust, faith, belief and expectation. Patterson (1967) indicated that there is some, but not much evidence that in the absence of these conditions, positive psychotherapeutic changes do occur (i.e., there are necessary conditions), but such evidence is limited to particular instances of the application of specific psychotherapeutic procedures and cannot be considered *the* necessary conditions for psychotherapy.

At the beginning of the chapter on situational analyses of the placebo effect, a definition of the placebo effect (Whitehorn 1968) was given; this definition, which places emphasis on expectational and relationship considerations, defines the placebo effect as ". . . all those psychological and psychophysiological benefits or determinants which quite directly involve the patient's expectations that depend directly upon the diminution or augmentation of the patient's apprehension by the symbolism of the medication or the symbolic implications of the physician's behavior and attitudes." Interestingly, in this definition psychotherapy also appears to depend directly upon the diminution or augmentation of the patient's apprehension by the symbolism (in the broadest sense of the word) of the physician's or psychotherapist's behavior and attitudes. In the preceding chapter we saw how important the patient's perception of such environmental and human interactional variables can be in the placebo effect. The position *in re* the necessary and sufficient conditions for the placebo effect appears to be essentially the same as those for psychotherapy: We can enumerate sufficient conditions but not necessary ones unless we call the necessary and sufficient condition the relationship between two people—that is, between the healer and the patient. Furthermore, the sufficient conditions for the placebo effect are, as we have seen in the research reviewed earlier, very similar to many of the sufficient conditions for psychotherapy: expectation, belief, trust in the doctor, attention, and, as Goldstein (1962) has indicated, a number of clear similarities between positive placebo reactors on the one hand, and therapy patients with favorable prognostic expectancies and those receptive to their therapists' expectancies, on the other. "For both placebo and psychotherapy patients of these types, anxiety level, degree of subjective distress, attraction to the therapist, [and] field dependence . . . appear to be important influences determining reaction to treatment. . . . in both instances we are examining individuals who are similar in several major respects" (Goldstein 1962, p. 110). Goldstein reviewed a number of studies conducted up to 1961, including one of his own (Goldstein and Shipman 1961). In a majority of the studies on the placebo effect in psychotherapy, Goldstein (1962) remarked,

much stress is placed on the proposition that the patient's reactions to the treatment procedures are in large part a function not of specific treatment effects, but of the more general influences stemming from: (1) the patient's need and desire to be helped, (2) the patient's expectation that such help will be forthcoming, (3) the performance, by the physician, of procedures associated in the patient's thinking with appropriate and effective treatment, (4) the performance of these procedures by a physician viewed by the patient as willing and able to provide help, and (5) the performance of these procedures in an institutional or related setting which is also associated by the patient with appropriate and effective treatment. In essence, we have described here the necessary and sufficient conditions of the placebo effect [pp. 104-05].

Goldstein stressed the placebo effect as a means of conceptualizing "spontaneous remission," as a prognostic device for predicting therapy outcome, and, very importantly, as an indicator of the quality of the therapist-patient relationship. It is also responsible for the "transference cure." In light of all these comments, is there a way in which we can be assured that psychotherapeutic intervention is more than merely placebogenic?

A superbly formulated answer to this question was provided by Rosenthal and Frank (1956) in a paper that has become one of the classics of the placebo literature. In order to show that a specific form of psychotherapeutic treatment produces more than a placebo effect, we have to show that its outcome is more effective, stronger, and of greater duration, than mere placebo treatment. There should also be qualitatively different effects for types of patients who would not be helped with placebos. The active agents that produce the desired results in psychotherapy are the theories of personality and psychotherapy to which psychotherapists adhere and according to which they plan their therapeutic actions. Unless there are controls for the placebo effect, there is no way of knowing whether effects predicted from a given theory of personality or psychotherapy lead to or result from improvement based on the placebo effect. Accordingly, Rosenthal and Frank (1956, p. 299) proposed that four conditions should be optimal in planning research in psychotherapy. First, a theory of personality and psychological distress should be used. (In behavior therapy, for example, this may not be a theory of personality per se as traditionally conceived, but it will certainly be a system of principles based on learning, reinforcement, and so forth. In our discussion, "theory of personality" should probably not be considered in its narrowest sense.) Second, we should, based on our theory or system, be able to predict effects in the patient as a consequence of psychotherapy. Third, some criterion of improvement is necessary, and a relationship between the criterion and the predicted effects needs to be shown. Fourth, we need to show as confidently as we can that the relationship between the predicted effects and the criterion is due to the specific techniques based on the theory or system, as opposed to merely the patient's belief or conviction that the theory will be of help. Thus we see that when a patient improves following a particular type of psychotherapy, such improvement cannot be viewed as evidence that the theory or system base is correct or that the specific technique is efficacious, "unless improvement can be shown to be greater than or qualitatively different from that produced by the patient's faith in the efficacy of the therapist and his techniques—'the placebo effect.' This effect may be quite powerful in that it may produce end-organ changes and relief from distress of considerable duration" (Rosenthal and Frank 1956, p. 300). A number of studies attempting to shed further light on just this aspect of the placebo effect will now be reviewed.

Kellner and Sheffield (1971) compared changes in distress scores following attendance at a clinic before and after treatment with changes in distress scores following subsequent brief interventions that were believed to have a therapeutic or suggestive effect: abreactions, brief psychotherapy, and a physical examination. The patients, all of whom were seen at an outpatient psychiatric clinic, had all suffered from neurotic reactions for at least the preceding six months. Group I consisted of anxious and depressed patients and Group II of hypochondriacal neurotics. Patients were told that they had to wait for treatment (the first waiting period). After this waiting period, Group I had three sessions of abreactions, consisting of intravenous thiopentone with methylamphetamine on alternate days, with each session lasting about forty-five minutes. The patients were told that the drug would make them feel drunk and drowsy and that the purpose was to help them talk freely about their problems and that what they said would be tape recorded and used as the topics for interviews. A second waiting period of the same duration as the first followed. Then the patients attended three therapy sessions on alternate days during which the tape recordings were played back to them and used for interpretive psychotherapy. After this, the Group I patients were told that they would have to wait for their followup treatment (third waiting period). Patients in Group II had a full physical examination with conventional X-ray and laboratory diagnostic procedures. After the results of these became available (about one week), the patients had one session with the therapist during which they were told that they were physically healthy and were given "explanatory therapy" regarding psychosomatic complaints. Patients were told that they would have to wait for their followup treatment (third waiting period). Fifteen patients completed the study, the results of which showed that the scores on the Symptom Rating Test administered every two weeks throughout the study decreased significantly during the first waiting period before treatment, but not during the other waiting periods.

This study confirmed the findings of previous studies that there is a substantial early improvement in distress scores, "probably due, in part, to the 'impact of a clinic' . . . or the 'response to the symbols of competent care'. . . . the present findings indicate that this effect can be greater than the effects of *subsequent* deliberate reassurance, suggestion, and brief psychotherapy" (Kellner and Sheffield 1971, p. 197). This study is a fine example of how early in the psychotherapeutic process placebo effects can manifest themselves. It also shows how, unless the criteria advanced by Rosenthal and Frank (1956) are utilized, the "psychotherapy" applied here was also a placebo. With regard to the early placebo effect exhibited, Hathaway's (1948) comments on the "hello-goodbye" pattern are of interest. When a patient starts off with a therapist, he or she meets the general cultural requirements for getting acquainted, which is a progression from initial greetings to eventual breaking off. The goodbye pattern includes changes in vocal intonation, tentative parting movements, and statements that tend to summarize. "Topics of conversation are implied to have been adequately treated and no new ones are brought up. . . . [there is a feeling of indebtedness and good will toward the therapist] not necessarily related to therapeutic outcomes but . . . likely to reflect a social interaction of the goodbye type" (Hathaway 1948, pp. 228-29). In addition, some patients, in trying to "save face," may not present safe issues rather than basic or really troubling ones at least until the "hello" period is concluded, so that the therapist may be misled into thinking that really significant improvement has occurred at the end of the first session. What Hathaway was describing sounds very much like the demand characteristics present early in psychotherapy, even though Orne's (1962) work on demand characteristics as such was not presented until a good two decades later. Therapists need to be aware that the discrepancy between the patient's expressed and actual relief after the first psychotherapy session may be far greater than we think it is or than we have measured it to be; hence the placebo effect of the first interview may not, in some cases, be as great as it appears to be at first glance. An interesting area of study would be to investigate the differences between relief of "serious" versus "superficial" problems following the initial psychotherapy interview, for one might hypothesize that in many cases the hello-goodbye pattern would bring about greater relief of the latter and less relief of the former types of problems. Some of the psychological factors involved in the relief following the first interview session were investigated in the next study to be examined here.

Goldstein and Shipman (1961) studied thirty neurotic outpatients in initial psychotherapy sessions. Three hypotheses were investigated. The first was that patients' expectations of symptom reduction due to psychotherapy is related positively and curvilinearly to perceived symptom reduction and positively and linearly to degree of patient pretherapy symptom intensity. The second hypothesis stated that the nature of the patient's referral for psychotherapy affects his or her pretherapy expectation of symptom reduction and pretherapy confidence in the clinic. The third hypothesis was that the degree of favorableness of the psychotherapist's attitudes toward psychotherapy and psychiatry is positively and linearly related to the degree of symptom reduction. The thirty therapists were all senior medical students seeing patients for psychotherapy as part of the psychiatry requirement of their medical curriculum. Patient expectation of symptom reduction was operationally defined as the difference between a patient's responses to a symptom-intensity inventory under "present-self" test-taking orientation and the patient's responses to the same inventory under "expected-self" orientation, with both sets of responses being obtained before the first therapy session. Patient-perceived symptom reduction was defined in operational terms as the difference between the patient's responses to a symptom-intensity inventory under "present-self" orientation prior to the first therapy and his or her responses to the same inventory under the same test-taking orientation immediately following the initial psychotherapeutic interview. Confidence in the clinic was operationally defined as the mean rank assigned to "clinic" by the patient when he or she was presented with a list of fifty common symptoms, each of which was followed by five alternative sources of help (friend, parent, no one, clinic, clergyman), and instructed to respond to each symptom statement by ranking the five possible sources of help in the order in which they would be recommended to a friend if the latter had given the complaint. Attitudes toward psychiatry and psychotherapy were operationally defined as the score obtained by the therapist on the Attitudes toward Psychiatry Scale, and nature of referral for psychotherapy was defined in terms of the assumption that people in mental health professions would be more likely than other possible referral sources to impart explicitly and implicitly favorable attitudes toward psychotherapy to their patients. Two groups of patients were classified: Those who had been referred by "favorable" referrals (psychiatrists, psychologists, social workers, and self-referrals) and "neutral" and "unfavorable" referrals (including general medical practitioners, nonpsychiatric medical specialists, parents, friends, and others).

The results of this study indicate that there is a significant curvilinear relationship between the degree to which the patients anticipate symptom reduction due to psychotherapy and the symptom reduction they perceive as taking place during the initial interview. Moderate patient expectation of therapeutic gain was associated with the greatest initial interview symptom reduction (at least according to the patient). There was also a significant linear relationship between pretherapy patient expectancy and the number and intensity of the symptoms the patients attributed to themselves before therapy. Goldstein and Shipman's study employed a correlational and not a causal analysis for this finding, but there is the suggestion of a motivational component in the patient's expectancy estimate insofar as the greater the degree of patient stress of discomfort, the greater his or her motivation for obtaining relief and, thus, the greater the expectancy that such relief would ensue. The results failed to support the hypothesized effect of referral source on expectancy, but there was a significant effect of referral source on confidence in the clinic. The authors suggested that the difference in responsiveness of these two patient characteristics to referral source may well have revolved around the multiplicity of determinants of individual expectancies. They quoted Rotter's (1954) statement that ". . . generalization, patterning, effects on expectancy of past experience, the unusualness of an occurrence, ambiguous cues, and so on, make up some of the variables that affect internal probability or expectancy" (p. 107). Confidence in the clinic may well have been less subject than expectancy to the variety of influences suggested by Rotter, thereby making the effect of referral source on confidence more clearly discernible.

The degree of favorableness of the therapist's attitudes toward psychiatry and psychotherapy was correlated with the degree of symptom reduction reported by the patient. A relationship between these variables was found (+0.387, significant at the .05 level) and appeared to be "yet another of the growing number of illustrations available in the literature of the significant relationship between therapist and patient characteristics in the psychotherapeutic interaction" (Goldstein and Shipman 1961, p. 133). This study is an important one since, by teasing out the nonspecific variables involved in the symptom reduction at the end of the first interview, the nature of the placebo effect was somewhat demystified; even when there is no active attempt to use therapeutic principles, significant patient relief can still be obtained.

Piper and Wogan (1970) conducted a study similar to that of Goldstein and Shipman, but instead of focusing on symptom reduction, they focused on change in affective states and extended the test-retest period to one week. The subjects were forty undergraduates seeking therapy from a university mental health clinic. The Multiple Affect Adjective Check List (MAACL), scored for the states of anxiety, depression, and hostility, was used as the measure of affective states, and the measure of expectancy was based on 130 items from the Mooney Problem Check List. When subjects came to the clinic for an initial interview, they were asked to complete the expectancy measure and the MAACL, and when they returned about a week later, the MAACL was again completed (but before the first therapy session). Between the first and second tests, there were significant decreases in the levels of anxiety, hostility, and depression and the total number of adjectives checked. However, correlation coefficients revealed no significant relationship between expectancy of improvement and change in any of the three affective states. The change in affective states was primarily due to checking fewer negatively toned adjectives while the number of positively toned adjectives remained about the same. The authors suggested the possibility that subjects actually felt better, that they reported less affect because they no longer needed to prove that they needed help, or that they were responding with a defensive response set. However, the data available did not permit a choice between these alternative explanations. On the basis of this study, therefore, and that of Goldstein and Shipman (1961), we have evidence that nonspecific effects can occur even before the initiation of psychotherapy per se. These effects can be changes in affective states and, in addition, in terms of measures of symptom reduction.

Leder (1969) reported on a number of studies conducted at a psychiatric clinic where patients with neurotic disorders stayed for eight weeks. They were treated by a combination of individual and group psychotherapy and were engaged in other activities such as occupational therapy and ward group meetings. In selected cases (not specified by the author, but never before the third week), patients received drugs. Symptom improvement in the first two weeks was what Leder (1969) described as "spectacular" (p. 115), particularly in the first week following admission. During the third week no further significant improvement was seen, and during the week before discharge, there was even some reappearance of symptoms. Leder explains these results as follows: The reduction of symptoms begins immediately after the patient has been admitted to the clinic, when a feeling of security results from the influence of various nonspecific factors in the therapeutic setting. These nonspecific factors meet the patient's needs for emotional contact and cognitive information. "This stage of passive learning merges with the next stage, which begins in the second or third week of [the patient's] stay, when the systematic planned application of therapeutic influencing in terms of a conceptual framework promotes active relearning and some of its results, namely insight and reorientation. Thus evaluation on discharge assesses changes which result from both passive learning—the placebo effect—and active relearning" (Leder 1969, p. 119). The psychotherapeutic process is thus conceived of as consisting of two stages: satisfaction of the needs of emotionally distressed patients for emotional contact and cognitive information, which constitutes the placebo effect, and then the achievement of other goals, with modifications occurring on a more integrated level. The placebo effect is an important part of the therapy; it is not an undesirable or unwanted embarrassment to the power of the therapy or the therapist. A similar process was suggested by Fish (1973) in his advocacy of capitalizing on the placebo effect in psychotherapy.

In Leder's study, the psychotherapy was not considered to be a placebo, but Campbell and Rosenbaum (1967) conducted a study where psychotherapy was viewed as being nothing but placebogenic. The initial sample for the study consisted of all patients newly assigned for treatment during a five-month period in a general psychiatry clinic. Prior to the first of two research interviews, each patient received a packet of materials to complete and bring in with him or her. The packet contained three documents: The Edwards Personal Preference Schedule, the Discomfort Scale, and a questionnaire that consisted solely of items reflecting the social and personal characteristics of the placebo reactor described in the literature. In the first research interview, which took place just before the first therapy session, patients were asked about presenting symptoms, distress, and social and personal characteristics, and these and diagnostic impressions were coded on a form. What was the placebo? As will be recalled, *placebo* was defined at the beginning of this book as "any therapeutic procedure (or that component of a therapeutic procedure) that is deliberately given to have an effect on, or does have an effect on, a symptom, syndrome, or disease, but that is without specific activity for a condition to be treated." As we have seen, things other than medications can have this effect, and Campbell and Rosenbaum (1967), remarking that "the findings in the literature provide the materials for testing a number of hypotheses asserting relationships between a patient's personality characteristics, initial distress, and relief of distress following a specified amount of psychotherapy," reasoned that from this paradigm, the placebo unit (according to the definition of placebo given above) was the first four weeks of psychotherapy and its context: "While such a definition may affect certain sensibilities, attempts to delineate specific factors in psychotherapy as responsible for improvement have for the most part failed, even though many reports of the efficacy of psychotherapy are to be found" (p. 365). A comment on such "sensibilities" will be made after we have examined the rest of Campbell and Rosenbaum's study.

Patients were ranked along three major scales: the P scale, reflecting the personality characteristics and attitudes ascribed to placebo reactors, the S scale, determining the degree of symptom stress the patients demonstrated at the first interview, and the R scale, measuring relief of symptoms after four weeks of psychotherapy. The P scale was derived from the work of Liberman (1964), who found that the placebo reactors described in his studies of drug-induced pain relief seemed to have many personality characteristics in common. The subjects were rated on the P scale, and divided into $P+$, P, and $P-$ groups; this rating was based on selected subscales of the Edwards Personal Preference Scale, a questionnaire, and an interview designed to assess patients on the personality characteristics of placebo reactors (e.g., regular church attendance, likes everybody, talkative, dependent, many somatic complaints under stress, takes aspirin and cathartics regularly, frequently diagnosed as anxious or depressed). Four subgroups were singled out on the basis of a natural clustering of certain traits that repeatedly have been reported to characterize placebo reactors. These subgroups were P-benevolent (sees self and others as benevolent, friendly, and helpful), P-religious (attends church regularly, feels religion is an important part of life), P-drug (frequently bothered by minor aches and pains and often uses nonprescription drugs), and P-gregarious (outgoing, friendly, one who seeks others' companionship regularly).

In the symptom distress groups, $S+$ and $S-$, symptoms were operationally defined using three instruments: a self-administered Discomfort Scale (a checklist composed of somatic and mental distress items rated on a five-point scale of severity), an interview to ascertain major or target symptoms ranked on a seven-point scale, and interviewer's judgment of patient's general symptomatic distress, also rated on a seven-point scale. Four symptom distress groups were obtained: target symptom distress, presenting symptom distress, somatic symptom distress, and mental symptom distress. The median overall symptom distress score was used to divide the study group into $S+$ and $S-$, high and low overall symptomatic distress, and high and low for each of the four symptom distress subgroups. All four measures of symptomatic distress were obtained again for each patient after four weeks in psychotherapy. The differences between the initial and four-week scores gave the symptom relief measures. Median split divided the study group into $R+$ and $R-$, high and low overall symptomatic relief, and the same method gave high and low symptomatic relief subgroups: target symptom relief, presenting symptom relief, somatic symptom relief, and mental symptom relief.

The authors report that four weeks of psychotherapy were conducted by eighteen psychiatric residents and clinic staff members (none of whom treated more than four patients), although the nature of the psychotherapy was not discussed by the authors. A followup interview was then conducted and symptom relief scores were collected. Six hypotheses were confirmed after examination of the data. First, $P+$ patients initially present more total symptomatic distress than do $P-$ patients. Second, $P+$ patients present a greater ratio of somatic distress to mental distress than do $P-$ patients. Third, patients with high initial distress report more relief of distress over four weeks of psychotherapy than those with low initial distress. Fourth, patients in the $P+$ group are older and have more formal education than those in the $P-$ group. Fifth, within the $P+$ group, the $P-$ drug subgroup shows significantly more distress and then relief of distress than any other group of patients. However, high initial distress is significantly correlated with high relief of symptoms regardless of P ranking. Sixth, patients presenting with predominantly mental symptoms demonstrate significant relief of those symptoms after four weeks of psychotherapy whereas those presenting predominantly somatic symptoms do not show such relief.

According to the authors, this experiment supported a major assumption from the literature, namely, that there is a group of patients who are placebo reactors. It also makes the important observation that patients with high initial distress will report more relief following psychotherapy than will those with low initial distress. This study is an interesting one; the measurement units chosen for analysis were ingenious, and the results might appear to be valid. However, the whole study flounders on the basis of one of the assumptions Campbell and Rosenbaum made: The placebo unit was the first four weeks of psychotherapy, even though, to quote the authors' statement cited earlier, "such a definition may affect certain sensibilities." Had the authors specified the type of therapeutic procedure used and had they even started to use Rosenthal and Frank's (1956) criteria for ascertaining that such therapy was not placebogenic, then we could rest assured that the treatment given consisted of even a little more than the mere nonspecific effects common to almost any therapeutic situation. However, since the type of therapy used in the study was not even named, the authors were not justified in assuming that the psychotherapy was a placebo, Rosenthal and Frank's criteria notwithstanding. The authors seem to have reasoned rather fallaciously that psychotherapy equals placebo, and this assumption is not warranted unless they felt their therapists' command of psychotherapy to have been such that all therapeutic changes were due to nonspecific influences. Clearly, in this case a psychotherapy placebo might not have been a placebo at all.

That a placebo component can exist even in such "scientific" treatments as systematic desensitization was demonstrated by McReynolds and Tori (1972) who investigated the influence of placebo and demand characteristics present in many comparisons of systematic desensitization and relaxation or attention-placebo treatments. The hypothesis tested was that systematic desensitization, presented (as it usually is) to subjects as an innovative and powerful therapy built on psychological and physiological principles that require concentrated involvement in a quasi-hypnotic setting, would create greater expectancy and demands of behavior than would relaxation treatment, which is less involving and less dramatic. The investigators predicted that desensitization would effect greater reductions in the target- (snake) avoidance behavior and reported fear but also on an ostensibly fear-related control task administered before and after treatment. This task, which subjects believed was a frustration tolerance test reflecting changes in fear and frustration, entailed fifteen minutes of crossing out twos and sixes on pages filled with random numbers, followed by ratings of felt frustration or aversion on a ten-point "frustration-aversion thermometer."

"Differential demand and placebo effects for [experimental] groups should be evident in differential pre-treatment-post-treatment changes in number of rows of numbers completed (performance control) and ratings of frustration-aversion (self-report control)" (McReynolds and Tori 1972, p. 262). Twenty-eight subjects were randomly assigned to one of three groups: systematic desensitization, relaxation treatment, or no treatment. Pretreatment-posttreatment changes revealed consistent improvements on both fear-related and control measures for the systematic desensitization group, while the relaxation group and the no-treatment group showed little or no change. The systematic desensitization group showed significantly greater gains than did the relaxation and no-treatment groups on the approach test, the frustration tolerance test, and the frustration-aversion thermometer. In addition, the systematic desensitization and relaxation groups showed greater reductions than did the no-treatment group on the fear thermometer.

These results suggest that systematic desensitization and relaxation treatments differ in the extent to which each generates subtle demands and expectancies of treatment-related behavior changes. On treatment-irrelevant control measures, subjects receiving systematic desensitization showed notable changes that tended to be correlated with other treatment-related behavior changes. McReynolds and Tori state that their results suggest that the superiority of systematic desensitization over relaxation treatments shown previously in the literature might not have been due to specific treatment procedure, but rather general behavior influences. One could say that the short nature of their treatment resulted in overemphasizing demand and placebo influences in comparison to real desensitization effects. But, on the other hand, longer treatment could make such effects even stronger. "Certainly the lack of substantiation of any other variable as *the* crucial ingredient in the desensitization process together with the present findings indicates a need for further investigation of placebo and related phenomena in desensitization" (McReynolds and Tori 1972, p. 263).

We shall now consider a different aspect of the placebo effect in psychotherapy, namely, the attempt to use placebo controls in studies of the effectiveness of psychotherapy. Only a few of the vast number of studies on psychotherapy process research will be included here, since the primary focus of this section is upon discussing the placebo aspects and not upon reviewing the literature on process research in psychotherapy. First, some of these studies will be examined with particular attention paid to the placebo controls used, and then some comments on these controls will be made.

Paul's (1966) factorial study of systematic desensitization was the first such study to be presented in the literature. It has become a classic in the field and praised, for example, by Yates (1970) who noted that "it has justly become celebrated" (p. 349). Paul compared systematic desensitization with traditional psychotherapeutic techniques in the treatment of public speaking anxiety in college students. After an extremely comprehensive pretreatment assessment procedure, subjects were assigned to three treatment groups, each of which was to receive individual systematic desensitization, insight-oriented psychotherapy, or attention placebo treatment. The fourth group was a nontreatment "waiting list" control, and the fifth group, a no-contact control. The attention placebo treatment required subjects to perform a vigilance task while under the influence of what they were told was a "fast-acting tranquilizer drug" (actually a placebo) that supposedly inhibited anxiety engendered by the task. The therapist gave them a good deal of nonspecific attention and support, the object of which was to control for the probable effects of attention, warmth, therapist interest, expectation of relief, suggestion, and faith. At the end of the treatment and at the first followup (Paul 1966) and two years later (Paul 1967), the systematic desensitization procedure was found to have been superior over all the other procedures; insight-oriented therapy and the placebo were not significantly different and both were superior to the no-treatment groups. In another study and followup (Paul 1968), group desensitization was found to be similarly successful.

Public speaking was treated by Trexler and Karst (1972) who compared the effects of rational-emotive therapy, placebo, and no treatment. Thirty-three college students reporting high levels of public speaking anxiety received rational-emotive therapy (RET), attention placebo, or no treatment. All subjects were mailed the Irrational Beliefs Test, based on Ellis' (1958) theory of psychopathology, and a modified version of Gilkinson's Personal Report of Confidence as a Speaker. Subjects were asked to bring the completed materials, along with a prepared speech on one of a number of suggested topics pertaining to their personal experience, to the first test-speech appointment, and just before giving their speech, each subject was asked to complete a fifteen-point anxiety scale. Treatment groups, matched approximately on the basis of the preliminary self-rating, were randomly assigned at the initial speech session.

Subjects in the no-treatment group were informed that there would be a short delay before they would begin therapy. For the others, there were four group sessions spaced several days apart. The RET group received therapy conducted largely along the lines proposed by Ellis. The attention placebo treatment, in which we are particularly interested here, consisted mainly of the typical training commonly used in systematic desensitization therapy, but without the construction and presentation of stimulus hierarchies. "The expectancy was communicated continually that this procedure was a well-regarded treatment for general anxiety and as such would be helpful in overcoming public speaking anxiety. Training was effected both with a recording and *viva voce*. Homework assignments for all sessions consisted of practicing relaxation skills and reading specially prepared materials . . . emphasizing both the purpose and techniques of relaxation" (Trexler and Karst 1972, p. 61). Primary analyses of pretherapy to posttherapy changes on the various measures tended to support the conclusion that RET was more effective than either the no-treatment or attention placebo treatment. Secondary analyses, which included the attention placebo and no-treatment subjects who received RET immediately after serving in those conditions, added further support for RET effects. (This study also hints that one person's systematic desensitization is almost another's placebo!)

Harris and Bruner (1971) attempted to assess the relative effectiveness of a self-control approach, a contract system, and an attention placebo control procedure on weight loss. The treatment period consisted of twelve weeks of regular weight checks during which the treatments were administered. The self-control procedure involved eight group meetings in which the rudiments of behavior theory (particularly operant and respondent conditioning) and their application were explained. For example, subjects selected punishment and other negative consequences for approaching food or for overeating, as well as positive reinforcement for both long-term and short-term goals. In the contract procedure, each subject made a cash deposit of xn and would receive it back at the rate of x per pound lost, the week after each pound's loss was recorded, until n pounds had been lost and all xn had been refunded. The contract also provided for forfeiture of the remaining dollars if the subject did not appear at the weekly weight check or notify the experimenter of cancellation, with the money to be divided equally among the remaining participants at the end of the twelve-week period. The attention placebo control group was told at the first meeting that treatment would consist of individual counseling and weekly weight checks. Pseudo-counseling consisted of the experimenter's passively listening to the subject's describing personal dieting problems, weight history, and related problems. Results indicated that both the contract and self-control groups lost a significant proportion of body weight between weeks one and twelve, with the weight loss after twelve weeks being significantly greater for the contract group than for either of the other two. A second experiment was conducted using only self-control and attention placebo groups for sixteen weeks, with no significant difference being exhibited at the end of this period between the two groups. In both studies, the "attention-placebo control group condition, involving information about nutrition, sympathetic listening, and a request for record-keeping did not accomplish any of the objectives" (Harris and Bruner 1971, p. 353).

Yet another placebo control was used in a study by Mosko (1972). The purpose of this research was to compare the efficacy of three treatment conditions for reducing withdrawal and promoting interpersonal relatedness among chronically hospitalized schizophrenics. The three treatments were physical contact therapy (PCT), verbal-oriented therapy (VOT), and an attention placebo control. Pre- and posttherapy measures of interpersonal functioning, withdrawal, concern for others, and general psychiatric adjustment were taken. Treatment consisted of twenty-one one-hour group sessions over a twenty-eight-day period. The results indicated that PCT produced a significant gain in the amount of concern a patient was willing to offer others and the length of time he or she would interact verbally with a stranger. On other variables, no-treatment condition was consistently superior to the other two, and overall treatment outcomes were more similar than different.

Sachs, Bean, and Morrow (1970) tested differential effects on smoking behavior of three treatments: covert sensitization, self-control, and attention placebo. Subjects' operant level of smoking was recorded for one week, after which random assignment to one of three groups was made. Each subject was seen four times: once for the assessment of operant level and three times for treatment procedures. On the last visit, subjects were instructed to continue the procedure and informed that they would be contacted by phone in one month for followup evaluation. The attention placebo condition involved subjects' being told that the increased awareness of their smoking patterns, as a function of continued careful recording of their smoking behavior, was an effective method of eliminating or reducing their cigarette consumption. The therapist collected and discussed subjects' smoking records throughout this treatment, with verbal approval provided for the completion of the records and for any of the subjects' statements of an increased awareness of their smoking patterns. The average duration of contact time between the subject and the therapist was ten minutes per session. The self-control condition involved the categorization of the initial week of smoking behavior into the relevant discriminative stimuli leading to smoking; ratings of the discriminative stimuli conditions according to the anticipated difficulty of not smoking in these stimulus situations were made, and subjects were instructed to discontinue smoking in the presence of the easiest situation. The covert sensitization involved the usual covert sensitization procedures, with pairing of pleasurable smoking scenes with aversive ones. Analysis of the results indicated significant smoking reduction over time. The best treatment results (mean number of cigarettes smoked per day) were found in the covert sensitization group, who smoked least, followed by the self-control group; the least effective treatment was the attention placebo condition, in which subjects smoked the most.

In the above studies (Paul 1966, 1967, 1968; Trexler and Karst 1972; Harris and Bruner 1971), the attention placebo conditions were all similar in that they involved some interaction between therapists and patients or subjects that was intended to create situations in which the patients (who were presumably rather naive in their knowledge of what constitutes psychotherapy) were supposed to think that they were undergoing actual psychotherapy. Insofar as these procedures involved no implementation of any known, specific therapeutic method, they were nonspecific. An examination of the literature on process and outcome research in psychotherapy reveals many similar attention placebo controls. For example, Paul (1969) reviewed fourteen controlled investigations of individual systematic desensitization, at least four of which involved the use of attention placebos. Such use is apparently widespread, but was the purpose for which attention placebos were used in the studies reviewed above such that they can be called "placebos"? While the attention placebos met the requirements of the definitions of "placebo" we have used in this book, the way in which such placebos were used forces us to consider the use of the word *placebo* to be an extremely unfortunate one in such circumstances and one that (unless we actually consult a particular study to see what the procedure was) is very misleading for several reasons.

In drug research, the placebo is usually *identical* in every observable way (especially when exact placebos are used) to the experimental substance being investigated. Particularly in double-blind studies, neither physician nor patient (nor others treating or evaluating) knows whether patients are receiving drug or placebo. Hence, all the personal interactions between the people involved are presumed to be identical for both groups. That this is not so in the case with the so-called attention placebos is ineluctably clear; indeed, such treatment conditions seem to maximize, rather than minimize, treatment interpersonal interaction differences. In one of the studies examined above, the authors (Sachs, Bean, and Morrow 1970) even stated that "the employment of therapeutic conditions necessitating unique procedural manipulations . . . were designed to maximize differences across treatment conditions" (p. 470).

Another very significant problem here is that the method is essentially single-blind. Since the therapists were all aware that the subjects in the so-called attention placebo conditions were not receiving the active treatment, the interaction could have been subject to all the pitfalls and biases inherent in any single-blind procedure. And to add even further to this complication, a double-blind method for evaluating psychotherapy is hardly conceivable unless either the therapist involved knows nothing about therapy, so that he or she will not know that a placebo is being used, or there is no therapist involved at all (a computer or tape recording could be the therapist, or could it, in the light of Truax's research, e.g., Truax and Mitchell, 1971)? And even then, how would one account, either qualitatively or quantitatively, for the placebo effects that might arise prior to therapy (e.g., in the pretherapy evaluation of the patient)?

What most researchers have been doing, therefore, is using attention *controls*, not attention *placebos*, and their data are not nearly as demonstrative of the difference between specific and nonspecific effects in psychotherapy as they might presume them to be. Their research relies for its evaluation not upon the measured effects of a presumed active psychotherapeutic procedure compared to those of something else, and this situation is so vastly different from that in drug research that the use of placebos in drug research cannot be considered to be analogous to psychotherapy placebos. Placebos are conceived of as offering the form, but not the substance, of treatment, and psychotherapy placebos, as conventionally used, do neither. Since a "psychotherapy placebo control" is an impossibility, we should talk of, for example, attention control groups in psychotherapy research, thereby appreciating the greater difference between experimental and control groups that this implies.

The term *psychotherapy placebo* should therefore be used only when we are talking of such nonspecific variables as hope, trust, and expectancy. These are factors that, as we have seen from our examination of the experimental literature, can be responsible for any placebo effect, be it in psychotherapeutic, drug, or any other form of treatment.

There are several methodological problems with placebo in research. The first is the problem concerning when and whether placebo effect really occur in particular subjects and situations where placebos are administered and where the second concerns problems associated with using placebos with pretesting.

9

Perspectives on Some Methodological Problems in Placebo Research

There are *with* *in*

Several methodological problems in placebo research have already been encountered in this book. We have seen, for example, the use of unstandardized tests of questionable reliability and validity, the failure to administer pretests so that the effects of treatment cannot be measured adequately, and subject acquiescence and consequent bias in the use of such instruments as symptom checklists. In this chapter we shall mention a number of less obvious but equally important problem areas. The first of these deals with problems concerning when and whether placebo effects really occur in particular subjects and situations where placebos are administered; the second concerns problems associated with pretesting; and the third deals with problems associated with the double-blind method.

We shall first look at problems concerning placebo effects in certain types of subjects and situations and the necessity for no-treatment controls. Davies (1964) has cautioned researchers to be aware of a kind of psychological event that can occur frequently in treatment, often remain undiscovered, and be mistaken for a placebo effect. Davies mentioned a patient whom he saw together with two other psychiatrists (so that the impressions of the patient were all based on the same interview material). All three psychiatrists were struck by sudden improvement in the patient. This improvement coincided with a change in the medication, and because of the absence of other identifiable factors, the psychiatrists assumed that the change in medication was the cause of the improvement. However, Davies (1964) indicated that "at a subsequent attendance the patient let slip the fact that his mother-in-law had died just as he began to improve. In view of the history which later emerged of the very bad relationship between himself and his mother-in-law, and the destructive effect she had had upon his household, we felt we could no longer ascribe his improvement to the drug but rather to his happy release" (p. 158). A problem like this one can be very real and can serve as a warning to researchers: Environmental contingencies may produce nontreatment effects that are ascribed to treatment, and this can happen more easily in the case of outpatients, over whose lives investigators have far less control, than in the case of inpatients.

Honigfeld (1968), too, has warned researchers to be aware of what he called "placebo reactions versus reactions during placebo treatment" (p. 98). Not all effects that occur during placebo treatment are placebo effects. For example, assessing the outcome of placebo treatment itself versus the spontaneous course of the disorder is often necessary, particularly in depressive disorders, because of

129

the spontaneous remission or cyclic course that many such disorders manifest. What might look like a placebo effect could be either a limited observation of part of a cycle that includes both manic and depressive episodes or a spontaneous symptom remission that is a part of the natural course of the disorder. One of the ways in which this problem could be handled is by considering the pill-giving ritual as an independent variable that is compared with a no-treatment control group.

Honigfeld has also mentioned how the absence of control groups can be a hindrance in the assessment of placebo effects in different diagnostic groups. In most depressive disorders, therapeutic response to placebo treatment follows a roughly normal distribution. In retarded depressions, the distribution tends, however, to be bimodal, which thus implies that there are really two subclassifications: patients who are not placebo responders and those who exhibit good response to placebo treatment. The latter group probably consists of two subgroups, in one of which the spontaneous course of the disorder is observed, while in the other there is a true placebo effect. Without a no-treatment control group, this finer subdivision cannot be made.

A number of studies examined in the preceding chapter showed that after the initial contact a patient has with a therapist, there can be a marked relief of distress even if this contact has involved only the administration of assessment instruments and so forth and no implementation of psychotherapeutic procedures per se. The fact that merely observing and changing environmental conditions for subjects can influence what is being measured and change its characteristics is well known, a famous example in psychology being the so-called Hawthorne effect. Roethlisberger and Dickson (1939) noticed this effect, and when various work conditions such as illumination, hours of work, wage rate, and so forth were manipulated in order to study the effects on production, they examined how production increased irrespective of the manipulation. They found the act of measuring changed not only the magnitude of the dependent variable but also the nature of the social situation. Workers felt important because they were chosen for the experiment, and feeling that they were members of a team, they worked together for the benefit of the team as a whole.

Psychological experiments are usually designed to test an hypothesis of change from an initial state of an organism to some other state as a result of an experimental treatment, necessitating the assessment of the preexperimental magnitude of a given variable. As Lana (1969) has indicated, although substituting a randomization design for a pretest design (so that any differences among the scores of the various groups are directly comparable to one another) is possible, a pretest will, given a constant n, often increase the precision of measurement by controlling for individual differences within subgroups. Should there be a failure of randomization, comparison of the subgroups' test measures will indicate this failure. Pretests are also administered to detect differences in initial performance so that the effects of some experimental manipulation taking into account these differences can be examined (as is the case in most placebo experiments). We know that in placebo studies the actions involved in measurement can affect the subject in some way. Any manipulation of the subject or of his or her environment by the experimenter prior to the treatment, which is to be followed by some measure of performance, allows for the possibility that the result is due either to the effect of the treatment or to the interaction of the treatment with the prior manipulation. An analysis of this kind of problem was made by Lana (1969) and will be modified here with particular reference to placebo experiments.

Suppose we are conducting an experiment to examine the effect of a week of placebo treatment on anxiety reduction in newly admitted hospitalized patients. Suppose, too, that we have strong suspicions, based on the kinds of evidence presented in the chapter on the placebo effect in psychotherapy that nonspecific effects involved in the pretreatment measurement will contribute to anxiety reduction. What design would we use? Four groups would be needed: Group I, the experimental group, would consist of patients given what is essentially prior manipulation—that is, a test such as the Taylor Manifest Anxiety Scale (MAS) to measure anxiety followed by one week of placebo treatment, at the end of which period the MAS would again be administered. Group II would be a control group that is given the MAS at the beginning and end of the week, without the placebo treatment. However, if we were to stop there, we would have no allowance for the evaluation of the effect of the treatment alone on the second MAS administration. A second control group (Group III) consisting of the placebo treatment followed by the measure of performance is therefore needed to allow the measurement of the effect of the treatment alone. One source of variation still remains unaccounted for, since conceivably the performance on retesting alone might be quite similar to performance under any or all of the conditions contained in Groups I and III. The fourth group, MAS alone, is therefore needed too.

Lana has pointed out that certain assumptions must be made concerning the distribution of the subjects in the four groups involved in this example: random sampling and random assignment to groups and an estimation of the comparability of the pretreatment measures for groups that cannot be pretested. If one can assume that there is a high probability that the un-pretested groups (i.e., III and IV) would not be significantly different from those who were pretested, then a 2 x 2 factorial analysis of variance can be computed on the posttest scores of the four groups. Finding a significant main effect for treatment indicates that the treatment affected the posttreatment score, as would be the case for a significant main effect. If, however, a significant interaction term is found, it should act as a warning device, and the use of the pretest would become suspect for the given data of the study.

Several cautions need to be associated with the use of a pretest. The subject may be aware of the manipulatory intent of the experimenter and the experimenter's expectations (cf. the experimenter effect). Also, the subject might be concerned about being evaluated. Campbell and Stanley (1966) have shown that a pretest may create an artificial "experiment participating effect" for the subject if the connections between pretests, treatment, and posttest are obvious. One way that this situation might be changed is by using equivalent forms of the particular instruments involved in the research. Lana (1969) commented on the substitution for the pretest of some other technique of observation or measurement of initial standing that "lacks the obvious and telltale characteristics of the pre-test" (p. 137). One might use unobtrusive measures, but Lana (1969) believes that the strongest impact of such measures on him "was to reinforce his belief in the necessity of looking for ways and devices to utilize reactive measures where the reaction (sensitization) on the part of the subject can either be measured or eliminated altogether" (p. 139). A design like the one in the example that has just been examined is useful in placebo research since it separates nonspecific placebo effects from the effects of the placebo itself. The design is not without its problems, but it does take us a long step further in ensuring a minimum of artifact in an area already laden with the possible confounding features of nonspecific effects.

The third problem area to be dealt with in this chapter concerns some aspects of the double-blind method. The use of a placebo control group in the use of a new compound, or the new application of an established one, is usually considered to be a sine qua non of clinical drug research. The usual assumption is that unless the double-blind is used, treatment effectiveness cannot be validly determined. "The double-blind condition in conjunction with randomization of subjects, precise assessment instruments, and appropriate statistical analyses provides, in contrast to the clinical trial approach, a degree of control over non-specific effects of treatment, i.e., personnel attitudes and expectancies, environmental influences and patient enthusiasm" (Guy, Gross, and Dennis 1967, p. 1505). Far from being a heaven-sent method, however, the double-blind is not infallible and consequently is not without its critics.

Tuteur (1958) maintains that when using the double-blind method, two drugs, the compound to be tested *and* the placebo (not just the compound to be tested), are being used. These may taste different, the side effects may be different, and the worsening of the patient's condition while on placebo may be demoralizing to both patients and personnel (as well as unethical). Constant and Dubois (1975) showed how such studies may have an important effect on personnel attitudes and their interactions with patients and how one cannot assume that in a double-blind study the only significant independent variables are active drug and placebo.

The problem of the different tastes of drug and placebo mentioned by Tuteur was also of interest to Blumenthal, Burke, and Shapiro (1974) who conducted a laboratory simulation of a double-blind clinical study in which inactive control drugs are described as "identical matching placebos." For the categories of minor tranquilizer, major tranquilizer, and antidepressant, subjects simulating experimenters or patients successfully differentiated active drugs from placebos based on physical characteristics of the medications. This study showed that many of the identical matching placebos could be differentiated from the actual drug in terms of such physical properties as texture, color, and thickness. These results suggest that comparisons of placebo and active drug should be made before a study begins, that administration of all medications (both active and placebo) should be in tasteless capsules, and that placebos should contain active ingredients to mimic the side effects of the active drug.

Cromie (1963) showed that the controls themselves may diminish the sensitivity of a trial, particularly when identical-appearing medications are used in a crossover trial. For example, a patient taking an analgesic tablet that makes him or her more comfortable at the beginning of a trial is liable to derive benefit from a placebo taken later if he or she thinks it is the same analgesic tablet. However, if the first tablet did not help, the patient might have negative expectations of the second one, thereby bringing the response to the two treatments closer together, decreasing the sensitivity of the trial, and making a distinction between the two agents less likely. Similarly, Batterman and Lower (1968), whose study we examined in the chapter on clinical uses of placebos, showed how the influence of previous therapy can persist for some time, so that part of what we might be seeing in so-called placebo or drug effects is partly such persistence. Batterman and Lower suggest that crossover evaluations of patients by double-blind methodologies seriously take into account the persistence of response to prior use of medications.

Barsa (1963) criticized the use of the double-blind method in the evaluation of tranquilizers. Tranquilizers have two separate and distinct actions: a sedative or calming action, which can be seen and measured relatively soon after the administration of the drug, and an antipsychotic action, which may only be detectable after several months. According to Barsa, in most double-blind studies the patients were kept on the drug for only a few weeks, and the subsequent effectiveness of the drug was its sedative action only, not its entire effectiveness, which thus led to false conclusions on the part of the investigators. In addition, the neglect of many researchers to take into account the individual dosage needs of a patient in their double-blind designs cannot give a valid picture of the effectiveness of a drug. Nash (1962) pointed out the necessity of distinguishing between the procedures employed and the results obtained, since the extent to which ideal double-blind conditions are actually approximated may, even with the application of identical procedures, vary from situation to situation. Parts of an experiment may actually be conducted in total or near-total blindness, while in other areas, the opposite may be the case. Ease of attainment of double-blind conditions is a function of the particular active medications and dosage levels being studied, the routes of administration of dosage forms employed, subjective effects of an oral dose (e.g., taste and texture of the medication and placebo), side effects, type of subjects, and the therapist-patient relationship.

Baker and Thorpe (1957) suggested that the persons making the observations in such experiments should remain naive in order to keep the experiment truly double-blind. This goal is, however, difficult to achieve since even if those observing and recording are not those who are treating, those treating may still obtain cues that break the blind and hence significantly affect interaction with the patient. Rosenthal (1963, cited by Guy, Gross, and Dennis 1967) concluded, on the basis of a number of experiments, that therapist bias might be eliminated by employing a third person as the data collector. The degree of bias would be reduced even if not entirely eliminated, particularly if the data collector is not prejudiced in the direction of the therapist's expectancies. Rosenthal emphasized that the failure of the double-blind method is not the failure of the "double-blindness" but rather of the maintenance of blindness, which may be threatened in close therapist-patient interactions. Other authors have even suggested that in the evaluation of antianxiety agents, single-organism paradigms be substituted as an alternative to conventional clinical trials using parallel groups (e.g., Uhlenhuth 1977). A free operant procedure was suggested. There have been many suggestions about eliminating double-blind procedures altogether.

Let us look, however, at a suggestion proposed by Guy, Gross, and Dennis (1967) that retains the double-blind procedure but with an important modification. In addition to the treating physician, these researchers employed an independent assessment team (IAT) consisting of a psychologist, a psychiatrist, and a social worker, each of whom was trained to rate specific treatment effects within the competency of his or her own professional discipline. "Lack of direct involvement in treatment reduces bias on the part of the IAT and produces a more objective appraisal of outcome" (Guy et al. 1967, p. 1506). Concurrent evaluations of approximately sixty patients were obtained by a daycare center psychiatrist and an IAT, and a significant difference was found to exist in the evaluation of treatment outcome between the psychiatrist and the IAT. The greatest mean discrepancy in rating occurred at pretreatment, with the patients being assessed as more disturbed by the psychiatrist than by the IAT. The discrepancy in diagnostic classification (psychotic versus nonpsychotic) was also significant, with the psychiatrist viewing more patients as psychotic than did the IAT. The psychiatrist was also, however, more optimistic as to treatment outcome, which may have led to bias in evaluating the outcome. Guy, Gross, and Dennis believe that the use of an IAT can prevent such occurrences by maintaining the objectivity of a double-blind procedure. This alternative refutes many of the criticisms of clinicians, contributes scientific rigor to a variety of evaluative problems for which the classical double-blind technique is either inapplicable or difficult to attain, and maintains the raison d'être of the double-blind procedure. The IAT concept can be superimposed directly on the double-blind procedure to add control over the problem of the inadvertent breaking of "blindness" by treatment personnel. When maintaining the "blindness" of the therapist is not possible, the IAT as well as the patient can remain blind. This technique allows the double-blind conditions to be verified instead of, as has so often been the case, merely assumed.

10 Some Further Theoretical Perspectives on the Placebo Effect

Looking at the placebo effect in great detail, we have seen the power it exerts in the large variety of situations in which it appears. In this chapter we shall simplify the role of theory by choosing perspectives that will allow the mass of data accumulated to date on the placebo effect to be tied together in meaningful ways. This review will permit not only a better conceptualization than exists at present of what we already know, but will also provide a sort of spring board from which hypotheses for future research may be derived. Some of these perspectives are not theories in the strictest sense of the word but rather general orientations within which the phenomena being considered can be viewed. They suggest the types of variables that need to be accounted for but are not all deductive systems from which clear, testable hypotheses can immediately be drawn. That few have been presented as explanations of the placebo effect per se is interesting; one of the striking characteristics of the literature on the placebo effect is that it is not theory based. One might look at this characteristic and say that it is not a fault, that the placebo effect, being a psychological phenomenon like any other psychological phenomenon, does not require any esoteric theory. I would agree with such a statement to some extent, but most of the studies reported in the literature have not even tested hypotheses derived from theories utilized in other areas of psychology.

As a consequence, systematic research efforts toward discovering the parameters of the placebo effect have been scant. The empirical studies, the experiments, and case reports that exist can make fascinating and often impressive reading, but one feels one is looking at pieces of colorful material that are awaiting cutting, trimming, and organizing before they can be made into an elegant quilt. Several of the investigatory studies reported have been poorly designed, unremarkable, and equivocal. Some have been what one of my professors once characterized as "*bubbe* psychology"—that is, they tell us no more about the problem than what our grandmothers (*bubbe* is the Yiddish word for "grandmother") would have been able to tell us without doing any research at all. In reading much of the literature on the placebo effect, one cannot help feeling that a large part of the research has been proceeding along what Hempel (1966) characterized as "the narrow inductivist conception of scientific inquiry." With little selection or a priori guesses as to their relative importance, large numbers of facts have been collected, analyzed (sometimes not), compared (sometimes), and classified (seldom), usually without hypotheses or postulates. Some generalizations have been made, but these have rarely been tested further. This situation is probably characteristic of early research in any area, but now that many preliminary investigations have been accomplished, the time might be right to be less empirical, to integrate what we know, to admit what we do not, and not to be afraid to use theory in a way that will allow us to further extend our hypothetical fingers since, orthodoxly speaking, empirical findings are logically relevant or irrelevant only in reference to a given hypothesis and not in reference of a given problem.

Marx (1963), in discussing the functions subsumed by theory, showed that most may be summarized by the statement that theory tends to be both an aid, sometimes perhaps an essential one, in directing empirical investigations (the tool function of theory) and also something valued as an objective in its own right (the goal function). The tool function of theory is what is immediately being called for in this chapter, for theories can guide research by generating new predictions not otherwise likely to occur. Marx cited Guthrie (1950) who said: "Systematic theory guides... observation and discovery. There are no raw facts" (p. 99). The goal function of theory suggests that theories order and integrate existing empirical laws, but since the empirical laws in placebo research cannot honestly be said to have attained such status, perhaps the heuristic results of the application of the tool function will allow the eventual strengthening of the aforementioned aspect of the goal function.

In a definition that would seem acceptable to most philosophers of science, Marx argued that there are three fundamental elements of all scientific theory construction or conceptual ordering of empirical data. These are, first, observations, which must be under controlled conditions; second, constructs, which must be operational, with clearly specified empirical referents; and third, hypotheses, which must be testable (i.e., clearly disconfirmable). The nature of most of the placebo literature published to date is empirical, with a consequent dearth of the third of these elements (i.e., hypotheses). Most of the explanations of the placebo effect that go one step beyond the data make use of such constructs as hope, faith, and expectancy, which are constructs that have not usually been clearly operationalized. These have already been encountered on numerous occasions throughout this book. No doubt such constructs are of great importance, and they appear in most current writing in the broad area of nonspecific effects. For example, Calestro (1972), wrote that "suggestibility, trust, and hope seem to be major factors in the outcome of any variety of therapeutic encounter, and the importance of these elements remains undistilled despite alterations in actual therapeutic technique" (p. 84). Our examination of the placebo literature has revealed how instructions can markedly affect the placebo effect and how therapists who are optimistic and confident can do the same thing, as can patient personality and a host of interactions between the patient and what Shapiro (1971a) called the "psychosociology of the physician." Such factors apparently facilitate change in a therapeutic context; faith or expectation for improvement, and not the "specific" validity of the actual treatment used (as long as what the healer does is consistent with the assumptive world of the patient), are where a large measure of the healing power lies. The first theoretical perspective to be encountered in this chapter is one that accommodates the most molar aspect of the placebo effect—hope and trust—and this presentation will be followed by perspectives that will allow the theoretical analysis to become narrower and more discrete.

The word *hope* might, at first hearing, sound like a taboo topic—that is, one of the untouchables with which psychology cannot or should not concern itself. But it is a word that figures prominently in the grander themes of human experience and is exemplified in such stock proverbs as "While there's life there's hope." It is a word that crops up repeatedly in literature and in the chronicles of human suffering. Shakespeare, in *Measure for Measure* (III, i), had Claudio say: "The miserable have no other medicine/But only hope," and Reid (1823), a prominent nineteenth-century physician, addressed its corollary (at least in the present usage of the word), faith, in a statement quite opposite to our present discussion when he said: "Faith will give a virtue to the most inefficient remedy; on the other hand, a distrust in the ability of a professional adviser will often defeat the tendency of his most judicious and seasonable prescription." Samuel Taylor Coleridge, in *Table Talk*, said: "He is the best physician who is the best inspirer of hope," and an old Irish proverb considers hope to be the physician of each misery.

One of the few psychologists to address this concept in a systematic way is Stotland (1969) who has pointed out that many psychologists avoid the use of subjective terms like "hope." Stotland proposed a framework within which to conceptualize hope by defining it largely in terms of expectations of things desired. In psychological terms, viewing hope as an expectation greater than zero of achieving a goal is useful. The degree of hopefulness thus becomes the level of such expectation, or the person's perceived probability of goal achievement. "It is therefore possible to integrate the definition of hope with approaches that use a concept of 'expectation' such as Tolman's (1948), Rotter's (1954), and Atkinson's (1964). *Hope* can therefore be regarded as a shorthand term for an expectation about goal attainment" (Stotland 1969, p. 2). Stotland has developed outlines for a theory concerning hopefulness levels and has attempted to apply this theory to experimental and field data in order to answer questions concerning causes and consequences of various levels of expectation of goal achievements. Of relevance to us here is Stotland's (1969) statement that the theory can be directed at "pointing out a necessary condition (albeit not a sufficient one) for therapy to be effective; that condition is hopefulness" (p. 5). Stotland has formulated a set of general propositions that are used to derive hypotheses by joining simple, plausible assumptions with a particular proposition, or by joining propositions, or by doing both. The theory was not formulated into an elegant axiomatic system, complete with axioms, implicit definitions, deductions, and operational definitions, for Stotland views the broaching of this less elegant type of theory as a necessary precondition for the emergence of a more elegant one.

Seven propositions are present in Stotland's theory. In the first proposition, the motivation for goal achievement is viewed partly as a function of the perceived probability of goal attainment and goal importance, with the goal being anything from food pellets to broad life goals, provided it is perceived or symbolized by the organism. Motivation refers to doing something (overt, covert, skeletal, perceptual, or cognitive behavior) as opposed to doing nothing. The second proposition involves affective states, so that positive affect will be experienced in proportion to the perceived probability of goal attainment and the importance of the goal. The third proposition involves anxiety arousal; there will be greater anxiety in proportion to how low the perceived probability of goal attainment becomes, and the relationship of this probability with goal importance. The truism that organisms are motivated to escape and avoid anxiety becomes the fourth proposition, with motivation becoming higher, the greater the anxiety experienced or expected. The first four propositions concern the level of expected probability of goal achievement. The necessary cognitive processes about relationships to goals are expressed in propositions five, six, and seven and involve schemas. These schemas are built of concepts and consist of associations between concepts. The fifth proposition tells us that schemas are acquired either through perception of a number of events in which examples of the same concepts are associated or through being communicated by other people. Schemas may be dormant or latent (not influencing action) or aroused (directly influencing action). Proposition six concerns the shift from dormancy to arousal that occurs when an event similar to a constituent part of the schema is perceived or when another person directs the person to invoke the schema. The schema is more likely to be aroused when there is strong similarity between the event and the constituent concept or when the person directing invocation of the schema is of importance to the person concerned. The last proposition, proposition seven, indicates that the strength and consistency of the schema, and the importance of the person from whom one acquired the schema, affect the probability that a schema will be invoked and remain aroused.

Hypotheses can be generated about the schemas that an organism develops about its own behavior, about its attainment of goals, about the effects other people have on goal attainment, about the relationships between schemas and anxiety, and so forth. Thus from the first proposition, we might hypothesize that the importance of the goal, and the expectation of achieving the goal, can lead to overt action toward the goal, covert symbolic action toward the goal, and selective attention to aspects of the environment relevant to attaining the goal. Essentially, this proposition considers hope to be a prerequisite for action, and in the case of the placebo effect, we would hypothesize that a patient's motivation to get well or experience symptom relief would be a positive function of the perceived probability of recovery and the perceived importance of recovery. The second proposition would allow us to hypothesize that the higher the perceived probability of recovery and the greater the importance of recovery, the greater will be the positive affect experienced by the patient. A patient's hopelessness about the important goal of recovery would, according to the third proposition, result in anxiety, which is a negative subjective state as well as a state of physiological arousal. The proposition implies that any perceived event that reduces the expectations of goal attainment will tend to increase anxiety. The fourth proposition would show that patients are motivated to escape and avoid anxiety, and a way in which this could be done would be through the schemas mentioned in the fifth proposition: The patient acquires schemas as a result either of his or her perception of a number of events in which examples of the same concepts are associated (e.g., a history of associating the administration of pills with the relief of distress) or of communication with other people (e.g., the physician telling the patient that symptom relief will follow the administration of whatever treatment is being used). The sixth proposition would indicate that communication from others can bring about invocations of the schema, thereby accounting for the ways in which instructions can affect the placebo effect. The greater the importance of the person directing the patient, the more likely the schema is to be aroused; from this we could test an hypothesis that, for example, the prestige of the physician will affect the magnitude of the placebo response experienced by the patient.

As Stotland (1969) has pointed out with regard to the way other people can influence schemas, communication is not the only relationship that can have such an influence. Mere perception of other people is also sufficient. Our perception of others is an event that occurs somewhere between communication from then and our perception of our own behavior. People's expectations, performance, and anxiety level can be influenced by their perception of other's expectations, performance, and anxiety just as they are influenced by perceptions of their own experiences. In the case of the placebo effect, research has shown that other people are not merely relevant to a person's expectations about his or her own actions: Their very actions may determine the person's potential for attaining his or her goals. A patient's anxiety level can be influenced by the perceived effectiveness of the physician or psychotherapist, and the patient can maintain a low level of anxiety just by being in the presence of a person who has been associated with goal attainment, which in this case is the process of becoming well. Stotland's theory could allow one to hypothesize that patients would strive harder to achieve symptom relief when others expect them to attain this than they would if there were no such expectation, and the power of such expectations is, in part, a function of the others' expertise and status. The other people could influence, direct, or even sometimes force the patient to act, and such action can then invoke a hopeful schema. Physicians can influence patients' hopefulness and anxiety by communicating, both verbally and nonverbally, positive expectations of their confidence that difficulties will be overcome. The power of the therapist's expectations in both medicine and psychotherapy is, of course, a well-established source of therapeutic influence.

Stotland's framework thus allows the implementation of an approach to studying the placebo effect that starts off with the most basic element, the patient coming for treatment, and allows the inclusion in a progressive way of more and more variables so that in a gradual and systematic way the complex picture of the whole placebo effect can be brought into focus, with each step following from the previous one. That such an approach is not simple is in part a function of the fact that the placebo effect is not a simple phenomenon; the framework of Stotland's psychology of hope permits the unfolding of the complex task of the operationalization of the psychological constituents of the construct of "hope" in the placebo effect in a systematic and fruitful way that has not been attempted to date.

At this point, theoretical perspectives from the psychology of learning can be brought into the discussion, since the rewarding qualities of discriminative stimuli and secondary reinforcements are similar to what Stotland talked about, particularly in the propositions involving schemas. Wilson, Hannon, and Evans (1968) remarked that the placebo effect is a reality and "an aspect of the subtle and often unwitting manipulation of the patient's behavior by the therapist, predictable from learning theory principles" (p. 105). Krasner (1962) interpreted the placebo effect as a generalized reinforcer, while Ullman and Krasner (1969) conceptualized the placebo itself as serving as a "discriminative stimulus because of its previous associations with curative agents" (p. 77), which is an approach criticized earlier in this book as being somewhat simplistic if one considers only the placebo itself, and not the whole context of its administration, as *the* discriminative stimulus.

The secondary reinforcement may be part of a hopeful schema—that is, it has usually been followed by the primary reinforcement. Mowrer (1960) presented an explanation of secondary reinforcement not at all incompatible with Stotland's psychology of hope. With particular reference to the placebo effect, Mowrer discussed this phenomenon as an example of "Secondary Reinforcement Type-2." In an earlier article he and Viek wrote (Mowrer and Viek 1948) we find:

One of the commonest yet most dramatic illustrations of this phenomenon is the relief experienced when the physician is consulted. One is ill and suffering from pain and inconvenience. The physician arrives, diagnoses the difficulty, prescribes treatment, and intimates that in a day or two one will be quite hale again. It is unlikely that the examination or the ensuing exchange of words has altered the *physical* condition of the patient in the least; yet he is likely to 'feel a lot better' as a result of the doctor's call. What obviously happens in such instances is that initially the patient's physical suffering is complicated by concern lest his suffering continue indefinitely or perhaps grow worse. After a reassuring diagnosis, this concern abates; and if, subsequently, the same ailment recurs, one can predict that it will arouse less apprehension than it did originally (provided, of course, that the physician's assurances were valid and his treatment effective) [p. 193].

Mowrer (1960) discussed "suggestion" in terms of learning theory and stated that this kind of suggestion is but another name for the effect produced by a type-2 secondary reinforcer; "it arouses hope or, equivalently, relieves apprehension and in so doing makes the individual *feel* better without, in a more fundamental sense, really *being* better" (p. 136). The essence of type-2 secondary reinforcement is that the onset of certain stimuli serve as "safety signals" eliciting the reduction of conditioned anxiety. "The cues producing decremental fear conditioning or hope in the therapeutic relationship would be the therapist's reassurances, his white coat, his title, etc., all part of culturally conditioned expectations of amelioration by entering professional care" (Wilson, Hannon, and Evans 1968, pp. 105-06).

The theoretical explanations of the placebo effect of Pavlovian conditioning (Herrnstein 1962; Hecht et al. 1968; Kissel and Barrucand 1967) mentioned elsewhere in this book can, of course, be partially subsumed under Mowrer's approach. Additional explanations along this line have been offered by Mathé (1966) and Meyer-Bisch (1967) among others. Meyer-Bisch noted that he was struck by "the similarities between the placebo effect and what Pavlov achieved with his dog: one can easily make the parallel between, on the one hand, the feeding of the dog and the sound of the bell, and, on the other, the medicinal substance and the context of its presentation. In both cases, the experimental findings appear to have shown that when one changes the substance but maintains certain aspects of its presentation, the reactions of the dog, like those of the patient, are the same" (p. 138, my translation). Mathé (1966) wrote:

Can we advance a specific theory of the mechanism of action of placebos? Yes, but it seems that the long period of study devoted to them leaves them still complex and obscure. The explanation given for the placebo effect can be either psychological, i.e. suggestion, or psychophysiological, i.e. conditioned reflex or stress. Anyway, for some people stress, when it exists, is an epiphenomenon and not a cause; the explanation for stress goes back to that of suggestibility. [Note: Mathé did not elaborate on his reasons for the latter statement.] Among the psychophysiological mechanisms for the placebo reaction, some are directly traceable to phenomena initiated by the taking of any medicine. These statements are extremely important, and we should refer to the work of Pavlov, Bykow and Selye . . . we should begin again, and use, in our clinics, the work of Pavlov [pp. 67-68, my translation].

An interesting way to account theoretically for Mowrer's (1960) statement that a placebo "makes the individual *feel* better without, in a more fundamental sense, *being* better" (p. 136) is by examining some relevant research on emotion. William James, in 1884, suggested that felt experience is subsequent to visceral discharge, that one feels bad because one has been crying and not vice-versa; "our feeling of [bodily] changes *is* the emotion." The cognitive components of the emotion were seen as the consequents to the perception of physiological change. In 1885, Carl Lange independently proposed a peripheral-origin theory sufficiently similar to James' version to be combined with it in later years; this theory is known as the James-Lange theory of emotion. W.B. Cannon presented a critical analysis of the relevant clinical and experimental literature on emotion and objected to the notion that the experience and expression of emotion is based on the perception of secondary sensations from the viscera (Grossman 1967). Cannon felt that emotions were central in origin and that their visceral components were unimportant in regulating emotional experience. The heart of the James-Lange versus Cannon controversy is the direction of the causal relationship between these factors. That direction may be irrelevant has been argued by Schachter (1964) who suggested that physiologically aroused subjects attach specific emotional labels to their arousal states that are consistent with concurrently experienced situational cues or cognitive factors. The person's perception of a link between cognitive and physiological factors rather than the actual existence of such a causal connection is crucial (Ross, Rodin, and Zimbardo 1969); contiguity between physiological arousal and emotionally relevant cognitive cues usually are sufficient to produce apparent emotion. I would apply Schachter's theory of emotion to the placebo effect in the following way: When people are in a state of arousal, they may experience very disparate emotional states or no emotional states at all, depending on the concurrent cognitions. This emotional plasticity leads people to search for cognitive sources that could be causally associated with their experienced physiological state and that could provide a label for it. A person taking a tablet, for example, is in a state of arousal (cf. Stotland's first and second propositions) and has learned to associate pill taking with relief of some sort (cf. the learning theory approaches outlined above). As a result of complex conditioning processes, visceral changes are initiated. These changes may be relatively undifferentiated physiologically and almost always take place contiguously with some set of cognitions (e.g., "This will make you feel better" or whatever the instructions, expectations of other communications or perceptions, tacit or not, in the schema are). The placebo effect can then, according to such a view, be interpreted as having three components: physiological arousal, emotionally relevant cognitive or situational factors, and a perceived causal link between these factors. A person who is not aware that he or she is being treated cannot exhibit the placebo effect; this is surely axiomatic.

The cognitive and situational factors mentioned in the Schachterian view, the labeling of patients' emotional states, and what we are told patients feel can all be related to recent work in the area of attribution research. In the study by Linton and Langs (1962) presented in the chapter on the personality of the placebo reactor, we saw that people who do not respond to placebos or who respond only weakly are introspective, alert, and sensitive to small differences and slight cues. Such people do not seem to rely on external situational factors to account for a perceived placebo effect. They do not *attribute* their internal states to extrapersonal cognitive and situational factors. The study by Weiner (1971), in our chapter on situational analyses of the placebo effect, showed how people would attribute psychological arousal to the placebo because they had been told that the placebo would produce such symptoms. The attributional process, involving how people explain the behavior of others and react to their own behavior, is becoming an increasingly important part of social psychological research. As Snyder (1976) said, "Research and theory in social perception and the attribution process are concerned with the processes by which individuals construct causal explanations for behavior and events. . . . the fundamental questions of one engaged in this information-processing task are . . . [whether] a particular sample of an individual's behavior [is] representative of corresponding inner states, dispositions or attitudes . . . or a reflection of current social and environmental pressures" (p. 56).

Few studies relating the placebo effect to attribution per se have been reported to date, probably because of the relative recency of the burgeoning of attribution research. That this is a promising area for placebo research was shown by Gibbons (1977). He hypothesized that objective self-awareness should reduce misattribution of arousal to a placebo. This hypothesis was partly based on previous research suggesting that awareness of internal dimensions is increased by self-focused attention and that in addition, the accuracy of causal attributions made about these states is increased as well. The subjects, female undergraduates, were placed in front of a mirror (either facing them and making them more self-aware, or facing away from them). Each was given a small packet of baking soda, either labeled as such or as "Cavanol," which they were told was a common laboratory drug with arousal properties similar to caffeine. Three arousal symptoms were ascribed to this "drug" for the subjects in the drug-misinformed condition: increased heart rate, sweaty palms, and a tightness in the chest. The symptoms would become noticeable three to four minutes after ingestion and would last about ten minutes. Each subject then was assigned an "observer" role to work on a task with a confederate of the experiment that required the subject's full attention. The task lasted seven and one-half minutes, following which two questionnaires were administered in succession. (Apparently no baseline measures had been taken.) The first questionnaire assessed perceptions of arousal level and reactions to the placebo, and the other was a sixteen-symptom checklist that included the three previously mentioned arousal symptoms and thirteen others.

The results showed that placebo ("Cavanol") subjects reported more arousal than baking soda subjects. Subjects who could see themselves in the mirror reported less arousal than those who could not. An interaction of self-awareness and drug was also shown. All subjects reported experiencing some arousal during the task. When asked "How aroused are you feeling right now?" (after the task was completed but before the alleged ten or so minutes of the "drug" effect had worn off), the arousal self-reports of the mirror subjects dropped off considerably after they stopped working on the task. This finding suggests that they attributed the arousal they were experiencing to the task and not to the placebo. In answer to the question "How arousing was the drug you took?" the self-aware subjects reported less drug-produced arousal. There was more arousal from the placebo than from the baking soda; self-aware subjects reported less drug-produced arousal than non-self-aware subjects; and the mirror had its primary effect in the placebo condition, where self-aware subjects reported much less drug arousal than did the non-self-aware ones. Regarding the salient symptoms, the non-self-aware group reported extremely high symptoms in comparison to the others.

Thus, Gibbons showed that self-focused subjects were not "fooled" by the placebo and had instead an accurate assessment of their reactions. This finding supported the hypothesis that awareness of arousal increases when attention is self-focused. The non-self-focused subjects were, however, placebo reactors who were attributing to the placebo the arousal produced by the experimental situation, as was corroborated by their high reports of symptom experiences. Although these subjects were not patients, this experiment does appear to be an excellent attempt to begin conceiving of factors involved in the placebo effect in relation to attribution. Of interest here is what we discovered in the personality chapter when looking at characteristics of patients who were placebo reactors. We saw them to be field dependent people with poor discrimination among medications, high acquiescence, and high symptom reporting. They react to cognitive suggestions with marked, subjectively perceivable psychological and physiological changes. The relationship of these characteristics with what Gibbons found is interesting and suggestive of the fact that attribution research could become an extremely fruitful base from which to conduct future research on the placebo effect. One need only think of how influential the therapeutic environment in general can be in order to see exactly why the concept of attribution is so useful here and relate Stotland's schemas to attribution in terms of the influence of the importance of communications and other people, as in propositions five, six, and seven. A network of interesting, testable hypotheses could be produced.

The application of theoretical perspectives such as those outlined above would allow greater operationalization of constructs that are often used in talking about the placebo effect. Consequent hypothesis testing would have great heuristic value. While there is no doubt that we are grappling with difficult conceptual problems, I think that these can be worked out better with theory than without. I am optimistic that the tool function in particular of the theoretical perspectives encountered here could well allow us to begin understanding far more about the placebo effect than we do now.

11 Overview and Coda

We have examined a number of perspectives on the placebo effect that range from what the patient brings to the therapeutic situation, through the type of treatment administered, to who the doctor is. Our review of the literature has pointed out that research on the physical aspects of the placebo itself has been quite inconclusive, that placebos can deal as effectively with a number of conditions such as anxiety and depression as can active drugs, and that the personality of the placebo reactor is not as unknown or as unknowable a variable as some writers would have us believe. We have also seen how important an influence the person of the doctor can be in the placebo effect, and how situational factors can be important determinants of the magnitude of the effect placebos can have. Clearly, the placebo effect is the product of the interaction between patient-personality-placebo-healer-situation variables, and because of this interaction, future research must be as inclusive as possible of such variables rather than parsimoniously one-sided.

I have made a plea for the abandonment of a totally empiricist approach to the study of the placebo effect and for the inclusion of theory-based research. Theory might well allow some trailing threads in current research to be gathered, and it would almost certainly usher in a surge of heurism in the study of the complex phenomena that make up the placebo effect. The fact that the phenomena are complex does not mean that they are not amenable to scientific study, and although the fact must be acknowledged that the total situation is not easily researchable, complexity should be neither a hindrance in planning further research nor an excuse for oversimplified approaches to the subject of study. There are still many questions to be asked and many answers to be found, but as Bronowski (1973) said, "We are always at the brink of the known" (p. 66) even if we have to revise some of our ideas and prejudices about science, its content, and its conduct.

This statement is particularly true when we turn back to the comments of Ellenberger (1970, p. 47) with which this book opened. After viewing Ellenberger's statements from the perspectives that have been presented on the placebo effect, we can see to what a large extent such a view of the difference between primitive and scientific therapy is idealized rather than actual. Primitive as well as modern healers are often the foremost personalities of their social group; both can exercise a great deal of their action primarily through their personalities, and both can be psychosomaticians, so that modern dichotomies between physical and psychic therapies are more posited than actual. Long and exacting training with much personal involvement is not the sole province of the primitive healer, for both primitive and modern healer frequently belong to schools that have their own teachings and traditions differing from those of other schools. Textbook medicine may be a branch of science and not an esoteric teaching; healing, the interface between therapist and patient, is not, but that does not mean that it cannot be investigated scientifically. The particular therapeutic models may vary, but modern healers are not vastly different *persons* from what they were eons ago. Diagnostic and therapeutic models must be consistent with the assumptive worlds of the cultures in which they are used, but functionally the healer and the patient are not playing different roles from those they have played throughout history.

The power of the placebo cannot fail to impress. This power is only mysterious insofar as the mysteriousness of human action can inspire a sense of wonder. The placebo effect attests to the power people can have, not in the sense of political might or coercion, but in the sense of overcoming personal adversity. Really understanding the placebo effect will allow us not to eliminate it from the realm of therapy but rather to use it so that all aspects of the therapeutic endeavor may benefit.

References

References

A Barefoot Doctor's Manual. 1977. Translation of Ch'ih chiao i sheng shou ts'e. Reprint of the 1974 edition published by the U.S. Department of Health, Education and Welfare. Philadelphia: Running Press.

Abramson, H.A., Jarvik, M.E., Levine, A., Kaufman, M.R., and Hirsch, M.W. 1955. LSD-25. XV. The effects produced by substitution of a tap water placebo. *Journal of Psychology* 40:367-83.

Adorno, T.W., Frenkel-Brunswik, E., Levinson, D.J., and Sanford, R.N. 1950. *The Authoritarian Personality.* New York: Harper.

Akiskal, H., and McKinney, W.T., Jr. 1973. Depressive disorders: Toward a unified hypothesis. *Science* 182:20-29.

American Psychiatric Association. 1968. *DSM-II: Diagnostic and Statistical Manual of Mental Disorders.* 2nd ed. Washington, D.C.

Appleton, W.S. 1971. Psychoactive drugs: A usage guide. *Diseases of the Nervous System* 32:607-16.

Atkinson, J.W. 1964. *An Introduction to Motivation.* New York: Van Nostrand.

Avorn, J. 1973. Beyond dying: Experiments using psychedelic drugs to ease the transition from life. *Harper's Magazine* (March):56-64.

Baker, A.A., and Thorpe, J.G. 1957. Placebo response. *Archives of Neurology and Psychiatry* 78:57-60.

Bank, S. 1969. An investigation of the placebo effect. *Dissertation Abstracts* 29 (7-B):2626.

Barber, T.X. 1969. *Hypnosis: A Scientific Approach.* New York: Van Nostrand, Reinhold.

————. 1970. *LSD, Marihuana, Yoga and Hypnosis.* Chicago: Aldine.

————, and Silver, M.J. 1968a. Fact, fiction, and the experimenter bias effect. *Psychological Bulletin Monograph* 70 (6, part 2):1-29.

————, and Silver, M.J. 1968b. Pitfalls in data analysis and interpretation: A reply to Rosenthal. *Psychological Bulletin Monograph* 70 (6, part 2):48-62.

Barsa, J.A. 1963. The fallacy of the "double blind." *American Journal of Psychiatry* 119:1174-75.

Batterman, R.C., and Lower, W.R. 1968. Placebo responsiveness—the influence of previous therapy. *Current Therapeutic Research* 10 (3):136-43.

Beecher, H.K. 1955. The powerful placebo. *Journal of the American Medical Association* 159:1602-06.

————. 1959. *Measurement of Subjective Responses: Quantitative Effects of Drugs.* New York: Oxford University Press.

————. 1961. Surgery as placebo. *Journal of the American Medical Association* 176:1102-07.

Bergersen, B., and Krug, E. 1969. *Pharmacology in Nursing.* St. Louis: Mosby.

Betz, B.J. 1963. Differential success rates of psychotherapists with "process" and "non-process" schizophrenic patients. *American Journal of Psychiatry* 119:1090-91.

Bishop, M.P., and Gallant, D.M. 1966. Observations of placebo response in chronic schizophrenic patients. *Archives of General Psychiatry* 14:497-503.

Black, A.A. 1966. Factors predisposing to a placebo response in new outpatients with anxiety states. *British Journal of Psychiatry* 112:557-67.

Blumenthal, D.S., Burke, R., and Shapiro, A.K. 1974. The validity of "identical matching placebos." *Archives of General Psychiatry* 31:214-15.

→ Braunstein, N.A., and Moscone, R.O. 1964. Consideraciones acerca la metodologia de la investigación psicofarmacológica. (Methodological considerations in psychopharmacological research). *Acta Psiquiátrica y Psicológica América Látina* 10:111-18.

Brodeur, D.W. 1965. The effects of stimulant and tranquilizer placebos on healthy subjects in a real-life situation. *Psychopharmacologia* 7:444-52.

Bronowski, J. 1973. The principle of tolerance. *The Atlantic* 232:60-66.

Brunswik, E. 1947. *Systematic and Representative Design of Psychological Experiments with Results in Physical and Social Perception.* Berkeley: University of California Press.

Butcher, J.N. (ed.). 1969. *MMPI: Research Developments and Clinical Applications.* New York: McGraw-Hill.

Caffey, E.M., Hollister, L.E., Kaim, S.C., and Pokorny, A.D. 1971. Drug treatment in psychiatry. *International Journal of Psychiatry* 9:428-71.

Calestro, K.M. 1972. Psychotherapy, faith healing and suggestion. *International Journal of Psychiatry* 10:83-113.

Campbell, D.T., and Stanley, J.C. 1966. *Experimental and Quasi-experimental Designs for Research.* Chicago: Rand McNally.

Campbell, J., and Rosenbaum, C.P. 1967. Placebo effect and symptom relief in psychotherapy. *Archives of General Psychiatry* 16:364-68.

Cannon, W.B. 1957. Voodoo death. *Psychosomatic Medicine* 19:182-90.

Carlson, R.J. 1975. A new paradigm? In R.J. Carlson (ed.), *The Frontiers of Science and Medicine.* London: Wildwood House.

Chapman, C.R., and Feather, B.W. 1973. Effects of diazepam on human pain tolerance and pain sensitivity. *Psychosomatic Medicine* 35:330-40.

Chomsky, N. 1968. Noam Chomsky and Stuart Hampshire discuss the study of language. *The Listener* 79:2044.

Claridge, G.S. 1961. The effects of meprobamate on the performance of a five-choice reaction-time task. *Journal of Mental Science* 107:590-602.

_____. 1972. *Drugs and Human Behavior.* Baltimore: Pelican.

Clark, W.C. 1967. The effect of an "analgesic" placebo on thermal sensitivity (d') and the criterion for pain. *Psychonomic Bulletin* 1 (2):8.

_____. 1969. Sensory-decision theory analysis of the placebo effect on the criterion for pain and thermal sensitivity (d'). *Journal of Abnormal Psychology* 74 (3):363-71.

Cofer, C.N., and Appley, M.H. 1964. *Motivation: Theory and Research.* New York: Wiley.

Cole, J.O., Bonato, R., and Goldberg, S. 1968. Nonspecific factors in the drug therapy of schizophrenic patients. In K. Rickels (ed.), *Nonspecific Factors in Drug Therapy.* Springfield, Ill.: Thomas.

Constant, J., and Dubois, J. 1975. Discours sur la methode double aveugle. *Revue de neuropsychiatrie infantile* 23:329-43.

Copi, I.M. 1961. *Introduction to Logic.* 2nd ed. New York: Macmillan.

Cowen, E.L. 1961. The experimental analogue: An approach to research in psychotherapy. *Psychological Reports* 8:9-10.

Cromie, B.W. 1963. The feet of clay of the double blind trial. *Lancet* 2:994-97.

Damarin, F., and Messick, S. 1965. *Response Styles as Personality Variables: A Theoretical Integration of Multivariate Research.* Princeton, N.J.: Educational Testing Service.

Davies, E.B. 1964. The problems of the placebo response. *Encéphale* 53:157-63.

Deutsch, M., and Krauss, R.M. 1965. *Theories in Social Psychology.* New York: Basic Books.

DiMascio, A. 1968. Personality and variability of response to psychotropic drugs: Relationship to "paradoxical effects." In Rickels (ed.), *Nonspecific Factors in Drug Therapy.*

_____, and Rinkel, M. 1963. Personality and drugs, "specific" or "nonspecific" influence on drug actions. In M. Rinkel (ed.), *Specific and Nonspecific Factors in Pharmacology.* New York: Philosophical Library.

_____, and Shader, R. (eds.). 1970. *Clinical Handbook of Psychopharmacology.* New York: Science House.

Dohrenwend, B., and Dohrenwend, B. (eds.). 1974. *Stressful Life Events: Their Nature and Effects.* New York: Wiley.

Duke, J.D. 1964. Placebo reactivity and tests of suggestibility. *Journal of Personality* 32 (2):227-35.

Eddy, N., and May, E.L. 1973. The search for a better analgesic. *Science* 181:407-14.

Ellenberger, H.F. 1970. *The Discovery of the Unconscious.* New York: Basic Books.

Ellis, A. 1958. Rational Psychotherapy. *Journal of General Psychology.* 59:35-49.

Ellis, A. 1959. Requisite conditions for basic personality change. *Journal of Consulting Psychology* 23:538.

Evans, F.J. 1967. Suggestibility in the normal waking state. *Psychological Bulletin* 67 (2):114-29.

_____. 1969. Placebo response: Relationship to suggestibility and hypnotizability. *Proceedings of the 77th Annual Convention of the American Psychological Association* 4 (part 2):889-90.

_____. 1974. The placebo response in pain reduction. In J.J. Bonica (ed.), *Pain. Advances in Neurology, 4.* New York: Raven Press.

Eysenck, H.J. 1967. *The Biological Basis of Personality*. Springfield, Ill.: Thomas.

_____, and Furneaux, W.D. 1945. Primary and secondary suggestibility: An experimental and statistical study. *Journal of Experimental Psychology* 35:485-503.

Farber, I.E. 1968. Personality and behavioral science. In M. Brodbeck (ed.), *Readings in the Philosophy of the Social Sciences*. New York: Macmillan.

Fast, G.J., and Fisher, S. 1971. The role of body attitudes and acquiescence in epinephrine and placebo effects. *Psychosomatic Medicine* 33 (1):63-84.

Fish, J. 1973. *Placebo Therapy*. San Francisco: Jossey-Bass.

Fisher, H.K., and Olin, B.M. 1956. The dynamics of placebo therapy: A clinical study. *American Journal of Medical Science* 232:504.

Fisher, S. 1967. The placebo reactor: Thesis, antithesis, synthesis and hypothesis. *Diseases of the Nervous System* 28:510-15.

_____. 1970a. Nonspecific factors in response to drugs. In DiMascio and Shader (eds.), *Clinical Handbook of Psychopharmacology*.

_____. 1970b. *Body Experience in Fantasy and Behavior*. New York: Appleton-Century-Crofts.

_____, and Fisher, R.L. 1963. Placebo response and acquiescence. *Psychopharmacologia* 4:298-301.

_____, and Fisher, R.L. 1964. Body image boundaries and patterns of body perceptions. *Journal of Abnormal Psychology* 68:255.

Forrer, G.R. 1960. Effect of oral activity on hallucinations. *Archives of General Psychiatry* 2:100-03.

_____. 1964. Psychoanalytic theory of placebo. *Diseases of the Nervous System* 25:655-61.

Frank, J.D. 1973. *Persuasion and Healing*. Baltimore: Johns Hopkins.

Frankenhaueser, M., Jaerpe, G., Svan, H., and Wrangsjoe, B. 1963. Psychophysiological reactions to two different placebo treatments. *Scandinavian Journal of Psychology* 4:245-50.

_____, Post, B., Hagdahl, R., and Wrangsjoe, B. 1964. Effects of a depressant drug as modified by experimentally-induced expectation. *Perceptual and Motor Skills* 18:513-22.

Fricke, B.G. 1957. A response-bias scale (B) for the MMPI. *Journal of Consulting Psychology* 21:149-53.

Gallimore, R.G., and Turner, J.L. 1977. Contemporary studies of placebo phenomena. In M.E. Jarvik (ed.), *Psychopharmacology in the Practice of Medicine*. New York: Appleton-Century-Crofts.

Gammer, C.E., and Allen, V.L. 1966. Note on use of drugs in psychological research. *Psychological Reports* 18 (2):654.

Garfinkel, H. 1967. *Studies in Ethnomethodology*. Englewood Cliffs, N.J.: Prentice-Hall.

Gartner, M.A. 1953. *Journal of the American Osteopathic Association* 60.

Gelfand, D.M., and Gelfand, S., and Rardin, M. 1965. Some personality factors associated with placebo responsivity. *Psychological Reports* 17 (2):555-62.

Gibbons, F.X. 1977. Self-focused attention and the attribution of arousal: Inhibition of the placebo effect. Paper presented at the 48th Annual Meeting of the Eastern Psychological Association, Boston, April 15.

Glass, L.B., and Barber, T.X. 1961. A note on hypnotic behavior, the definition of the situation, and the placebo effect. *Journal of Nervous and Mental Diseases* 132:539-41.

Glick, B.S. 1967. Placebo as prognosticator. *Diseases of the Nervous System* 28 (11):737-43.

Goldman, A., Witton, K., and Scherer, J.M. 1965. The drug-giving ritual, verbal instructions, and schizophrenics' ward activity levels. *Journal of Nervous and Mental Diseases* 140 (4):272-79.

Goldstein, A.P. 1962. *Therapist-Patient Expectancies in Psychotherapy.* New York: Macmillan.

_____, and Shipman, W.G. 1961. Patient expectancies, symptom reduction and aspects of the initial psychotherapeutic interview. *Journal of Clinical Psychology* 17:129-33.

Gowdey, C.W., Hamilton, J.T., and Philp, R.B. 1967. A controlled clinical trial using placebos in normal subjects: A teaching exercise. *Canadian Medical Association Journal* 96:1317-22.

Grossman, S.P. 1967. *A Textbook of Physiological Psychology.* New York: Wiley.

Guthrie, E.R. 1950. The Status of Systematic Psychology. *American Psychologist* 5:97-101.

Guy, W.H. 1967. Placebo proneness: Its relationship to environmental influences and personality traits. *Dissertation Abstracts* 28 (5-B):2137-38.

_____, Gross, M., and Dennis, H. 1967. An alternative to the double blind procedure. *American Journal of Psychiatry* 123:1505-12.

Haas, H., Fink, H., and Härtfelder, G. 1959. Das Placebo Problem. *Fortschritte der Arzneimittelforschung* 1:279-454.

Haertzen, C., and Hill, H.E. 1959. Effects of morphine and pentobarbital on differential MMPI profiles. *Journal of Clinical Psychology* 75:434-37.

Hall, A.R., and Hall, M.B. 1964. *A Brief History of Science.* New York: Signet.

Halm, J. 1968. The relationship of field articulation and affective placebo reaction. *Dissertation Abstracts* 28 (10-B):4283-84.

Hankoff, L.D., Freedman, N., and Engelhardt, D.M. 1958. The prognostic value of the placebo response. *American Journal of Psychiatry* 115 (6):549-50.

_____, Freedman, N., and Engelhardt, D.M. 1960. Placebo response in schizophrenic outpatients. *Archives of General Psychiatry* 2:33-42.

Harris, M.B., and Bruner, C.G. 1971. A comparison of a self-control and a contract procedure for weight control. *Behavior Research and Therapy* 9:347-54.

Harrison, T. 1963. The doctor's task. In H.I. Lief, V.G. Lief, and N.R. Lief (eds.), *The Psychological Basis of Medical Practice*. New York: Harper & Row.

Hathaway, S.R. 1948. Some considerations relative to nondirective counseling as therapy. *Journal of Clinical Psychology* 4:226-31.

Hecht, K., Hecht, T., and Treptow, K. 1968. Beziehungen zwischen Funktions-zustand des ZNS und dem Konditionierten pharmakologischen Effekt: ein Beitrag zum Placebo-Effekt. *Acta Biologica Medica Germanicae* 20:773-85.

Hekimian, L.J., and Friedhoff, A.J. 1967. A controlled study of placebo, chlordiazepoxide, and chlorpromazine with 30 male schizophrenic patients. *Diseases of the Nervous System* 28 (10):675-78.

Hempel, C.G. 1966. *Philosophy of Natural Science*. Englewood Cliffs, N.J.: Prentice-Hall.

Herrnstein, R.J. 1962. Placebo effect in the rat. *Science* 138:677-78.

Hochman, J.S., and Brill, N.Q. Marijuana intoxication: Pharmacological and psychological factors. *Diseases of the Nervous System.* 32:677-78.

Honigfeld, G. 1964a. Nonspecific factors in treatment: I. Review of placebo reactions and placebo reactors. *Diseases of the Nervous System* 25:145-56.

_____. 1964b. Nonspecific factors in treatment: II. Review of social-psycho-logical factors. *Diseases of the Nervous System* 25:225-39.

_____. 1968. Specific and nonspecific factors in the treatment of depressed states. In Rickels (ed.), *Nonspecific Factors in Drug Therapy*.

Horvath, L.G. 1965. *Psychological Abstracts* 39:105 (Abstract #937).

Imber, S.D., Frank, J.D., Gliedman, L.H., Nash, E.H., and Stone, A.R. 1956. Suggestibility, social class, and the acceptance of psychotherapy. *Journal of Clinical Psychology* 12:341-44.

James, W. 1901. *The Varieties of Religious Experience*. New York: Random House.

Joyce, C.R.B. 1959. A study of consistent placebo reactions. *British Journal of Pharmacology and Chemotherapy* 14:512-21.

Kasl, S., and Cobb, S. 1966a. Health behavior, illness behavior and sick-role behavior: I. Health and illness behavior. *Archives of Environmental Health* 12:246-66.

_____, and Cobb, S. 1966b. Health behavior, illness behavior, and sick-role behavior: II. Sick-role behavior. *Archives of Environmental Health* 12:531-41.

Kellner, R., and Sheffield, B.F. 1971. The relief of distress following attendance at a clinic. *British Journal of Psychiatry* 118:195-98.

Kissel, P., and Barrucand, D. 1964. *Placebos et effet placebo en médecine*. Paris: Masson.

_____, and Barrucand, D. 1967. La placébothérapie conditionèe sous hyp-nose. *Annales Médico-Psychologiques* 1 (4):579-85.

Knowles, J.B., and Lucas, C.J. 1960, Experimental studies of the placebo response. *Journal of Mental Science* 106:231-40.

Kornetsky, C., and Humphries, O. 1957. Relationship between effects of a number of centrally acting drugs and personality. *AMA Archives of Neurology and Psychiatry* 77:325-27.

Krasner, L. 1962. The therapist as a social reinforcement machine. In H.H. Strupp and L. Luborsky (eds.), *Research in Psychotherapy.* Volume 2. Washington, D.C.: American Psychological Association, pp. 61-94.

Kudlien, F. 1976. Medicine as a "liberal art" and the question of the physician's income. *Journal of the History of Medicine and Allied Sciences* 31:448-59.

Kurland, A.A. 1958. The placebo. In J.H. Masserman, and J.L. Moreno (eds.), *Progress in Psychotherapy.* Vol. 3. New York: Grune and Stratton.

Lana, R.E. 1969. Pretest sensitization. In R. Rosenthal and R. Rosnow (eds.), *Artifact in Behavioral Research.* New York: Academic Press.

Lang, W.J., and Rand, M.J. 1969. A placebo response as a conditional reflex to glyceryl trinitrate. *Medical Journal of Australia* 1, (3 May):912-14.

Lasagna, L. 1963. The relation of drug-induced changes to personality. In Rinkel (ed.), *Specific and Nonspecific Factors in Psychopharmacology.*

_____, Laties, V.G., and Dohan, L.J. 1958. Further studies on the "pharmacology" of placebo administration. *Journal of Clinical Investigation* 37:533.

_____, Mosteller, F., von Felsinger, J.M., and Beecher, H.K. 1954. A study of the placebo response. *American Journal of Medicine* 16:770-79.

Leder, S. 1969. Psychotherapy: Placebo effect and/or learning? *International Psychiatry Clinics* 6:114-33.

Lehmann, H.E., and Knight, M.A. 1960. Placebo-proneness and placebo-resistance of different psychological functions. *Psychiatric Quarterly* 34:505-16.

Liberman, R. 1964. An experimental study of the placebo response under three different situations of pain. *Journal of Psychiatric Research* 2 (4):223-46.

Linton, H.B., and Langs, R.J. 1962. Placebo reactions in a study of LSD-25. *Archives of General Psychiatry* 6:369-83.

Lipowski, Z.J. 1969. Psychosocial aspects of disease. *Annals of Internal Medicine* 71:1197-206.

_____(ed.). 1972. *Advances in Psychosomatic Medicine, Vol. 8: Psychosocial Aspects of Physical Illness.* Basel: S. Karger.

Lowinger, P., and Dobie, S. 1969. What makes the placebo work? A study of placebo response rates. *Archives of General Psychiatry* 20 (1):84-88.

Maher, B. 1966. *Principles of Psychopathology.* New York: McGraw-Hill.

Majno, G. 1975. *The Healing Hand: Man and Wound in the Ancient World.* Cambridge, Mass.: Harvard University Press.

Malitz, S., and Kanzler, M. 1971. Are antidepressants better than placebo? *American Journal of Psychiatry* 127:1605-11.

Marx, M.H. 1963. The general nature of theory construction. In M.M. Marx (ed.), *Theories in Contemporary Psychology.* New York: Collier-Macmillan.

Mathé, A. 1966. Le médecin, le malade et le médicament. *Revue de Médecine Psychosomatique* 8:65-69.

McGlashan, T.H., Evans, F.J., and Orne, M.T. 1969. The nature of hypnotic analgesia and placebo response to experimental pain. *Psychosomatic Medicine* 31:227-46.

McNair, D., Kahn, R., Droppleman, L., and Fisher, S. 1968. Patient acquiescence and drug effects. In Rickels (ed.), *Nonspecific Factors in Drug Therapy.*

McNemar, Q. 1946. Opinion-attitude methodology. *Psychological Bulletin* 43:289-374.

McReynolds, W.T., and Tori, C. 1972. A further assessment of attention-placebo effects and demand characteristics in studies of systematic desensitization. *Journal of Consulting and Clinical Psychology* 38:261-64.

Mechanic, D. 1972. Social psychologic factors affecting the presentation of bodily complaints. *New England Journal of Medicine* 286:1132-39.

Meehl, P.E. 1973. The Cognitive activity of the clinician. In P.E. Meehl, *Psychodiagnosis, Selected Papers.* Minneapolis: University of Minnesota Press.

Melzack, R. 1973. *The Puzzle of Pain.* Baltimore: Penguin.

_____ and Torgerson, W.S. 1971. On the language of pain. *Anesthesiology* 34:50.

_____, and Wall, P.D. 1965. Pain mechanisms: A new theory. *Science* 150:971.

Meyer, R.E. 1970. Treatment of alcoholism and drug addiction. In DiMascio and Shader (eds.), *Clinical Handbook of Psychopharmacology.*

Meyer-Bisch, R. 1967. Réflexions sur le probléme des placebos and de leurs méthodes d'application. *Annales de Therapeutique Psychiatrique* 3:138-43.

Moos, R. (ed.). 1977. *Coping with Physical Illness.* New York: Plenum.

Morris, L., and O'Neal, E. 1974. Drug-name familiarity and the placebo effect. *Journal of Clinical Psychology* 30:280-82.

Mowrer, O.H. 1960. *Learning Theory and Behavior.* New York: Wiley.

_____, and Viek, P. 1948. An experimental analogue of fear from a sense of helplessness. *Journal of Abnormal and Social Psychology* 83:193-200.

Mosko, A.F. 1972. A comparison of physical contact psychotherapy, verbal-oriented psychotherapy, and an attention-placebo control with chronically hospitalized schizophrenic patients. *Dissertation Abstracts International* 32 (7-B):4222-23.

Muller, B.P. 1965. Personality of placebo reactors and nonreactors. *Diseases of the Nervous System* 26:58-61.

Nash, H. 1962. The double blind procedure: Rationale and empirical evaluation. *Journal of Nervous and Mental Diseases* 134:34-37.

Orne, M.T. 1962. On the social psychology of the psychological experiment, with particular reference to demand characteristics and their implications. *American Psychologist* 17:776-83.

_____. 1970. Hypnosis, motivation, and the ecological validity of the psychological experiment. In W.J. Arnold and M.M. Page (eds.), *Nebraska Symposium on Motivation.* Lincoln: University of Nebraska Press.

Park, L.C., and Covi, L. 1965. Nonblind placebo trial. *Archives of General Psychiatry* 12 (4):336-45.

Patterson, C.H. 1967. Divergence and convergence in psychotherapy. *American Journal of Psychotherapy* 21:4-17.

Paul, G.L. 1966. *Insight versus Desensitization in Psychotherapy: An Experiment in Anxiety Reduction.* Stanford: Stanford University Press.

_____. 1967. Insight versus desensitization in psychotherapy two years after termination. *Journal of Consulting Psychology* 31:333-48.

_____. 1968. Two-year follow-up of systematic desensitization in therapy groups. *Journal of Abnormal Psychology* 73:119-30.

_____. 1969. Outcome of systematic desensitization. II: Controlled investigations of individual treatment, technique variations, and current status. In C.M. Franks (ed.), *Behavior Therapy: Appraisal and Status.* New York: McGraw-Hill.

Pichot, P., and Perse, J. 1968. Placebo effects as response set. In Rickels (ed.), *Nonspecific Factors in Drug Therapy.*

Pihl, R.O., and Altman, J. 1971. An experimental analysis of the placebo effect. *Journal of Clinical Pharmacology* 11:91-95.

Piper, W.E., and Wogan, M. 1970. Placebo effect in psychotherapy: An extension of earlier findings. *Journal of Consulting and Clinical Psychology* 34:447.

Pollak, K., and Underwood, E.A. 1968. *The Healers: The Doctor Then and Now.* London: Nelson.

Pomeranz, D.M., and Krasner, L. 1969. Effect of a placebo on a simple motor response. *Perceptual and Motor Skills* 28 (1):15-18.

Reid, J. 1823. *Essays on Hypochondriasis and Other Nervous Affections.* London: Longman, Hunt, Rees, Orne and Brown.

Richter, C.P. 1957. On the phenomenon of sudden death in animals and man. *Psychosomatic Medicine* 19:191-98.

Rickels, K. (ed.). 968a. *Nonspecific Factors in Drug Therapy.* Springfield, Ill.: Thomas.

_____. 1968b. Nonspecific factors in drug therapy of neurotic patients. In Rickels (ed.), *Nonspecific Factors in Drug Therapy.*

_____, and Downing, R. 1965. Verbal ability (intelligence) and improvement in drug therapy of neurotic patients. *Journal of New Drugs* 5:303-07.

_____, Cattell, R.B., Weise, C., Gray, B., Yee, R., Mallin, A., and Aaronson, H.G. 1966. Controlled psychopharmacological research in private practice. *Psychopharmacologia* 9:288-306.

_____, Lipman, R., and Raab, E. Previous medication, duration of illness and placebo response. *Journal of Nervous and Mental Diseases* 142 (6):548-54.

Rinkel, M. (ed.). 1963. *Specific and Nonspecific Factors in Psychopharmacology.* New York: Philosophical Library.

Roethlisberger, F.J., and Dickson, W.J. 1939. *Management and the worker.* Cambridge, Mass.: Harvard University Press.

Rogers, C.R. 1957. The necessary and sufficient conditions of therapeutic personality change. *Journal of Consulting Psychology* 21:95.

Rosenthal, D., and Frank, J. 1956. Psychotherapy and the placebo effect. *Psychological Bulletin* 53 (4):294-302.

Rosenthal, R. 1963. On the social psychiatry of the psychological experiment. *American Scientist* 51:268-83.

_____ and Rosnow, R. 1969. The volunteer subject. In R. Rosenthal, and R. Rosnow (eds.), *Artifact in Behavioral Research.* New York: Academic Press.

Ross, L., Rodin, J., and Zimbardo, P.G. 1969. Toward an attribution therapy: The reduction of fear through induced cognitive-emotional misattribution. *Journal of Personality and Social Psychology* 12:279-88.

Rotter, J.B. 1954. *Social Learning and Clinical Psychology.* Englewood Cliffs, N.J.: Prentice-Hall.

Sachs, L.B., Bean, H., and Morrow, J.E. 1970. Comparison of smoking treatments. *Behavior Therapy* 1:465-72.

Sarason, I.G., and Smith, R.E. 1971. Personality. *Annual Review of Psychology* 22:393-446.

Schachter, S. 1964. The interaction of cognitive and physiological determinants of emotional state. In L. Berkowitz (ed.), *Advances in experimental social psychology.* Vol. 1. New York: Academic Press.

Schimlek, F. 1950. *Medicine versus Witchcraft.* Marianhill, Natal, South Africa: Marianhill Mission Press.

Schofield, W. 1964. *Psychotherapy: The Purchase of Friendship.* Englewood Cliffs, N.J.: Prentice-Hall.

Selye, H. 1956. *The Stress of Life.* New York: McGraw-Hill.

Shader, R.I. 1970. Antianxiety agents: A clinical perspective. In DiMascio and Shader (eds.), *Clinical Handbook of Psychopharmacology.*

Shapiro, A.K. 1959. The placebo effect in the history of medical treatment: Implications for psychiatry. *American Journal of Psychiatry* 116:298-304.

_____. 1960. Contribution to the history of the placebo effect. *Behavioral Science* 5:109-35.

_____. 1963. Psychological use of medication. In H.I. Lief, V.F. Lief, and N.R. Lief (eds.), *Psychological Basis of Medical Practice.* New York: Harper & Row.

_____. 1964a. A historic and heuristic definition of the placebo. *Psychiatry* 27 (1):52-58.

_____. 1964b. Iatroplacebogenics. Paper presented at the American Psychiatric Association, Divisional Meeting, Philadelphia, November 24.

_____. 1966. The curative waters and warm poultices of psychotherapy. *Psychosomatics* 7:21-23.

_____. 1971a. The placebo response. In J.G. Howells (ed.), *Modern Perspectives in World Psychiatry: 2.* Edinburgh: Oliver and Boyd.

_____. 1971b. Placebo effects in medicine, psychotherapy and psychoanalysis. In A.E. Bergin and S.L. Garfield (eds.), *Handbook of Psychotherapy and Behavior Change.* New York: Wiley.

_____ , Wilensky, H., and Struening, E.L. 1968. Study of the placebo effect with a placebo test. *Comprehensive Psychiatry* 9 (2):118-37.

Sharp, H.C. 1965. Identifying placebo-reactors. *Journal of Psychology* 60 (2):205-12.

Smart, R.G., and Bateman, K. 1967. Unfavorable reactions to LSD: A review and analysis of the available case reports. *Canadian Medical Association Journal* 97:1214-21.

Snyder, M. 1976. Attribution and behavior: Social perception and social causation. In J. Harvey, W. Ickes, and R. Kidd (eds.), *New Directions in Attribution Research.* Vol. 1. Hillsdale, N.J.: Erlbaum.

Staehelin, J.E. 1960. Nichtalkoholische Suchte. *Psychiatrie der Gegenwart.* Band II. Berlin, Springer:340-68.

Steinbook, R.M., and Jones, M.B., and Ainslie, J.D. 1965. Suggestibility and the placebo response. *Journal of Nervous and Mental Diseases* 140 (1):87-91.

Steinhauer, P., Mushin, D., and Rae-Grant, Q. 1974. Psychological aspects of chronic illness. *Pediatric Clinics of North America* 21:825-40.

Sternbach, R.A. 1964. The effects of instructional sets on autonomic responsivity. *Psychophysiology* 1:67-72.

_____ . 1968. *Pain: A Psychophysiological Analysis.* New York: Academic Press.

Stotland, E. 1969. *The Psychology of Hope.* San Francisco: Jossey-Bass.

Strassman, H.D., Adams, B., and Pearson, A.W. 1970. Metronidazole effect on social drinkers. *Quarterly Journal of Studies on Alcohol* 31:394-98.

Tellegen, A. 1970. Some comments on Barber's "reconceptualization" of hypnosis. *Journal of Experimental Research in Personality* 4:259-67.

Thomas, T.R., and Hull, J.H. 1971. Effect of an anesthetic placebo on two-point thresholds. *Perceptual and Motor Skills* 32:235-38.

Thorn, Wendy Fairfax. 1962. The placebo reactor. *Australasian Journal of Pharmacy* 43:1035-37.

Thornwald, J. 1962. *Science and Secrets of Early Medicine.* New York: Harcourt, Brace and World.

Tolman, E.C. 1948. Cognitive maps in rats and men. *Psychological Review* 55:189-208.

Trexler, L.D., and Karst, T.O. 1972. Rational-emotive therapy, placebo, and no-treatment effects on public-speaking anxiety. *Journal of Abnormal Psychology* 79:60-67.

Trouton, D.S. 1957. Placebos and their psychological effects. *Journal of Mental Science* 103:344-54.

Truax, C.B., and Mitchell, K.M. 1971. Research on certain therapist interpersonal skills in relation to process and outcome. In A. Bergin and S. Garfield (eds.), *Handbook of Psychotherapy and Behavior Change.* New York: Wiley.

Tuteur, W. 1958. The "double blind" method: Its pitfalls and fallacies. *American Journal of Psychiatry* 114:921-22.

Uhlenhuth, E., Canter, A., Neustadt, J., and Payson, H. 1959. The symptomatic relief of anxiety with meprobamate, phenobarbital and placebo. *American Journal of Psychiatry* 115:905-10.

Uhlenhuth, E. 1977. Evaluating antianxiety agents in humans: Experimental paradigms. *American Journal of Psychiatry* 134:659-62.

Ullman, L., and Krasner, L. 1969. *A Psychological Approach to Abnormal Behavior.* Englewood Cliffs, N.J.: Prentice-Hall.

Vinar, O. 1968. A discussion of the appropriateness of placebo use in psychotic subjects. In Rickels, (ed.), *Nonspecific Factors in Drug Therapy.*

———. 1969. Dependence on a placebo: A case report. *British Journal of Psychiatry* 115:1189-90.

Watkins, J.G. 1963. Hypnosis. In N.L. Farberow (ed.), *Taboo Topics.* New York: Atherton Press.

Weiner, M.J. 1971. Contiguity of placebo administration and misattribution. *Perceptual and Motor Skills* 33:1271-80.

Welsh, G.S. 1956. Factor dimensions A and R. In G.S. Welsh, and W.G. Dahlstrom, (eds.), *Basic Readings on the MMPI in Psychology and Medicine.* Minneapolis: University of Minnesota Press.

Wheatley, D. 1968. Effects of doctors' and patients' attitudes and other factors on response to drugs. In Rickels (ed.), *Nonspecific Factors in Drug Therapy.*

Whitehorn, J.C. 1958. Psychiatric Implications of the placebo effect. *American Journal of Psychiatry* 114:662-64.

Wilson, G.T., Hannon, A., and Evans, W.I.M. 1968. Behavior therapy and the therapist-patient relationship. *Journal of Consulting and Clinical Psychology* 32 (2):103-09.

Wolberg, L.R. 1967. *The Technique of Psychotherapy.* New York: Grune and Stratton.

Wolf, S., and Wolff, H.G. 1943. *Human Gastric Function. An Experimental Study of Man and His Stomach.* London: Oxford University Press.

Yalovoy, A. 1969. A substitute for the alcohol-antabuse test in treating alcoholism with placebos. *Soviet Neurology and Psychiatry* 3:59-65.

Yates, A.J. 1970. *Behavior Therapy.* New York: Wiley.

Zegans, L.S., Pollard, J.C., and Brown, D. 1967. The effects of LSD-25 on creativity and tolerance to regression. *Archives of General Psychiatry* 16:740-49.

Zvonikov, M.Z. 1969. A modification of the technique for conditional reflex therapy of alcoholism based on apomorphine and suggestion. *Soviet Neurology and Psychiatry* 3:66-71.

Zweig, S. 1966. *Die Heilung durch den Geistes.* Frankfurt am Main: Fischer Verlag. (Originally published, Leipzig: Insel Verlag, 1931.)

Author Index

Aaronson, H.G., 106-107
Abramson, H.A., 22-23, 74, 76, 89
Adams, B., 52
Adorno, T.W., 80
Ainslie, J.D., 78, 90
Akiskal, H., 47
Allen, V.L., 12
Altman, J., 18-19
Appleton, W.S., 54
Appley, M.H., 37, 38
Atkinson, J.W., 139
Avorn, J., 24

Baker, A.A., 134
Bank, S., 94-96
Barber, T.X., 19, 22, 23, 51, 77, 88
Barrucand, D., xiv, xvi, 11-12, 13, 14,
    42, 53, 56, 87-88, 143
Barsa, J.A., 133
Bateman, K., 51
Batterman, R.C., 42, 133
Bean, H., 125, 126
Beecher, H.K., xv, 3, 26, 27, 28, 31,
    32, 36, 70-74, 90
Bergersen, B., 26, 28
Bishop, M.P., 44-45, 46
Black, A.A., 50
Blumenthal, D.S., 132-133
Bonato, R., 45-46
Braunstein, N.A., 41-42
Brill, N.Q., 25
Brodeur, D.W., 42, 96-97
Bronowski, J., 147
Brown, D., 23
Bruner, C.G., 124, 125
Brunswik, E., 39
Burke, R., 132-133
Butcher, J.N., 63

Caffey, E.M., 47
Calestro, K.M., 138
Campbell, D.T., 132
Campbell, J., 119-121

Cannon, W.B., 38, 143-144
Canter, A., 105-106
Cattell, R.B., 106-107
Chapman, C.R., 29
Chomsky, N., 7-8
Claridge, G.S., 21, 41, 47, 60, 77
Clark, W.C., 28
Cobb, S., 35, 38
Cofer, C.N., 37, 38
Cole, J.O., 45-46
Coleridge, Samuel Taylor, 139
Constant, J., 132
Copi, I.M., 111-112
Covi, L., 99-100
Cromie, B.W., 133

Damarin, F., 80
Davies, E.B., 129
Dennis, H., 132, 134-135
Deutsch, M., xvi
Dickson, W.J., 130
DiMascio, A., 68
Dobie, S., 45, 46, 102-103
Dohan, L.J., xv
Dohrenwend, B. and B., 37
Downing, R., 87, 90
Droppleman, L., 82-85, 86, 87, 90
Dryden, John, 25
Dubois, J., 132
Duke, J.D., 78-79, 90

Eddy, N., 26
Ellenberger, H.F., xi, 15, 19, 106,
    147
Ellis, A., 112, 123
Engelhardt, D.M., 45, 46, 53
Evans, F.J., 26, 28, 29-30, 31, 77-78,
    79, 88
Evans, W.I.M., 142, 143
Eysenck, H.J., 70, 77, 78, 91

Farber, I.E., 39
Fast, G.J., 85-86, 87, 89

Feather, B.W., 29
Felsinger, von, J.M., xv, 70-74, 90
Fink, H., 42
Fish, J., 119
Fisher, H.K., 60
Fisher, R.L., 79-80, 84, 85, 86, 89
Fisher, S., xiii, xiv, 8, 43, 61, 79-80, 82-86, 87, 89, 90, 91
Forrer, G.R., 3, 9-10, 12
Frank, J., 35, 79, 113-114, 115, 121
Frankenhaueser, M., 98
Freedmen, N., 45, 46, 53
Frenkel-Brunswik, E., 80
Fricke, B.G., 81
Friedhoff, A.J., 45, 46
Furneaux, W.D., 77

Gallant, D.M., 44-45, 46
Gallimore, R.G., 3, 90
Gammer, C.E., 12
Garfinkel, H., 39
Gartner, M.A., 89
Gelfand, D.M. and S., 28, 64-65, 89
Gibbons, F.X., 145-146
Glaser and Whittow, 12
Glass, L.B., 88
Glick, B.S., 53
Gliedman, L.H., 79
Goldberg, S., 45-46
Goldman, A., 13, 44
Goldstein, A.P., 93, 96, 104, 113, 116-117
Gowdey, C.W., 12, 20-21, 42
Gray, B., 106-107
Gross, M., 132, 134-135
Guthrie, E.R., 138
Guy, W.H., 67, 69, 89, 96, 132, 134, 135

Haas, H., 42
Haertzen, C., 63-64
Hagdahl, R., 98
Hall, A.R. and M.B., 5, 6
Halm, J., 66-67
Hamilton, J.T., 12, 20-21, 42
Hankoff, L.D., 45, 46, 53
Hannon, A., 142, 143

Harris, M.B., 124, 125
Harrison, T., 1, 6, 43
Härtfelder, G., 42
Hathaway, S.R., 115-116
Hecht, K. and T., 17-18, 19, 143
Hekimian, L.J., 45, 46
Hempel, C.G., 137
Herrnstein, R.J., 17, 18, 19, 143
Hill, H.E., 63-64
Hirsch, M.W., 22-23, 74, 76, 89
Hochman, J.S., 25
Hollister, L.E., 47
Honigfeld, G., xv, 12, 13, 14, 36, 47-48, 60, 89, 129-130
Horvath, L.G., 96
Hull, J.H., 97, 99
Humphries, O., 68

Imber, S.D., 79

Jaerpe, G., 98
James, William, 76, 143
Jarvik, M.E., 22-23, 74, 76, 89
Jones, M.B., 78, 90
Joyce, C.R.B., 64, 89

Kahn, R., 82-85, 86, 87, 90
Kaim, S.C., 47
Kenzler, M., 48-49
Karst, T.O., 123-124, 125
Kasl, S., 35, 38
Kaufman, M.R., 22-23, 74, 76, 89
Kellner, R., 114-115
Kissel, P., xiv, xvi, 11-12, 13, 14, 42, 53, 56, 87-88, 143
Klein et al., 48
Knight, M.A., 21-22
Knowles, J.B., 68-69, 89
Kornetsky, C., 68
Krasner, L., 11, 13, 21, 142
Krauss, R.M., xvi
Krug, E., 26, 28
Kurland, A.A., 60

Lana, R.E., 130-132
Lang, W.J., 19-20
Lange, Carl, 143

Langs, R.J., 23-24, 65-66, 89, 144
Lasagna, L., xv, 12, 13, 68, 70-74, 90
Laties, V.G., xv
Leder, S., 118-119
Lehmann, H.E., 21-22
Levine, A., 22-23, 74, 76, 89
Levinson, D.J., 80
Liberman, R., 119-120
Linton, H.B., 23-24, 65-66, 89, 144
Lipman, R., 54-56, 108
Lipowski, Z.J., 36-37
Lower, W.R., 42, 133
Lowinger, P., 45, 46, 102-103
Lucas, C.J., 68-69, 89

McGlashan, T.H., 29-30, 89
McKinney, W.T., Jr., 47
McNair, D., 82-85, 86, 87, 90
McNemar, Q., 63
McReynolds, W.T., 121-122
Maher, B., 14, 39
Majno, G., 6
Malitz, S., 48-49
Mallin, A., 106-107
Marx, M.H., 138
Mathé, A., 143
May, E.L., 26
Mechanic, D., 37
Meehl, P.E., 109
Melzack, R., 26, 27
Messick, S., 80
Meyer, R.E., 50
Meyer-Bisch, R., 7, 143
Mitchell, K.M., 111, 126
Moos, R., 37
Morison et al., 13
Morris, L., 99
Morrow, J.E., 125, 126
Moscone, R.O., 41-42
Mosko, A.F., 124-125
Mosteller, F., xv, 70-74, 90
Mowrer, O.H., 142-143
Muchin, D., 37
Muller, B.P., 62-63, 89

Nash, E.H., 79
Nash, H., 133-134

Neustadt, J., 105-106

Olin, B.M., 60
O'Neal, E., 99
Orne, M.T., 29-30, 39-40, 93-94, 115-116

Park, L.C., 99-100
Patterson, C.H., 110-111, 112
Paul, G.L., 122-123, 125
Payson, H., 105-106
Pearson, A.W., 52
Perse, J., 80-82, 89
Philp, R.B., 12, 20-21, 42
Pichot, P., 80-82, 89
Pihl, R.O., 18-19
Piper, W.E., 117-118
Pokorny, A.D., 47
Pollard, J.C., 23
Pomeranz, D.M., 21
Post, B., 98

Raab, E., 54-56, 108
Rae-Grant, Q., 37
Rand, M.J., 19-20
Rardin, M., 28, 64-65
Reid, J., 139
Richter, C.P., 38, 90
Rickels, K., xv, xvi, 54-56, 70, 74-75, 87, 90, 106-107, 108
Rinkel, M., xv, xvi, 68
Rodin, J., 144
Roethlisberger, F.J., 130
Rogers, C.R., 112
Rosenbaum, C.P., 119-121
Rosenthal, D., 113-114, 115, 121
Rosenthal, R., 63, 104, 134
Rosnow, R., 63
Ross, L., 144
Rotter, J.B., 117, 139

Sachs, L.B., 125, 126
Sanford, R.N., 80
Sarason, I.G., 91
Schachter, S., 90, 100, 102, 144
Scherer, J.M., 13, 44
Schimlek, F., 4

Schofield, W., 109
Selye, H., 37
Shader, R.I., 50
Shakespeare, 139
Shapiro, A.K., xiii, xv, 3, 6, 7, 53-54, 75, 89, 90, 103-105, 132-133, 138
Sharp, H.C., 64, 89
Sheffield, B.F., 114-115
Shipman, W.G., 113, 116-117
Silver, M.J., 19
Smart, R.G., 51
Smith, R.E., 91
Snyder, M., 145
Staehelin, J.E., 44
Stanley, J.C., 132
Steinbook, R.M., 78, 90
Steinhauer, P., 37
Sternbach, R.A., 29, 32, 98
Stone, E.H., 79
Stotland, E., 139-142, 144, 146
Strassman, H.D., 52
Struening, E.L., 53-54, 75
Svan, H., 98

Tellegen, A., 77
Thomas, T.R., 97, 99
Thorn, W.F., 29, 69-70, 89
Thorpe, J.G., 134
Tolman, E.C., 139
Torgerson, W.S., 27
Tori, C., 121-122
Traut and Passarelli, 13, 14
Treptow, K., 17-18, 19
Trexler, L.D., 123-124, 125
Trouton, D.S., 73-74

Truax, C.B., 111, 126
Turner, J.L., 3, 90
Tuteur, W., 132

Uhlenhuth, E., 105-106, 134
Ullman, L., 11, 13, 142

Valins, 101
Viek, P., 142
Vinar, O., xv, 44, 46, 49
Virchow, 6

Wainwright, 49
Watkins, J.G., 7
Weiner, M.J., 101-102, 144
Weise, C., 106-107
Welsh, G.S., 81
Wheatley, D., 107-108
Whitehorn, J.C., 94, 102, 112
Wilensky, H., 53-54, 75
Wilson, G.T., 142, 143
Witton, K., 13, 44
Wogan, M., 117-118
Wolberg, L.R., 109-110
Wolf, S., 41
Wolff, H.G., 41
Wrangsjoe, B., 98

Yalovoy, A., 51
Yates, A.J., 122
Yee, R., 106-107

Zegans, L.S., 23
Zimbardo, P.G., 144
Zvonikov, M.Z., 51-52
Zweig, Stefan, 1, 90

Subject Index

Acetophenazine, 45
Acquiescence, 79-87
Acupuncture and pulse doctrine, 4
Addiction, xv, 44
Advances in Psychosomatic Medicine
    (Lipowski), 36
Affective states, changes in, 118
African medicine, 4
Alcoholism, 50-52
Amylobarbitone, 107-108
Analgesia, 25-33, 64
Anesthetics, 26
"Anginine," 19
Animal studies, 17-19
Annual Review of Psychology, 91
Antabuse, 51
Antianginal drugs, 19
Antianxiety drugs, 70, 74
Antidepressant drugs, 48-49
Anxiety, 32, 50, 69-70, 107-108; trait/
    state, 29, 30
Apomorphine, 51
Arousal: physiological/psychological,
    100-102, 144-145; self-awareness,
    145-146
Arthritis, 42
Asclepius, 2
Aspirin, 11, 13, 26, 31
"Athletic"/"aesthetic" types, 68
Attention controls, 126
Attention placebos, 123-127
Attribution research, 144-146
Authoritarian Personality (Adorno et
    al.), 80
Autosuggestion, 42
Awareness of arousal, 145-146

Baking soda, 145-146
Barefoot Doctor's Manual, 5
Benactyzine, 18
Bernreuter scale, 64
Bias, experimental, 104, 134
Burn injuries, 32

Cannabis sativa, 24-25
Carryover effects, xv
"Cavanol," 145-146
Childbirth, 26-27
Chinese medicine, 4-5
Chlordiazepoxide, 45, 55, 70, 74, 81,
    107-108
Chloroform, 26
Chlorpromazine, 18, 44, 45, 46
Codeine, 31
Compliance, 75
Conditioning, 10-11, 17-20, 87, 124,
    143
Conditions, necessary/sufficient, 111-
    112, 113
Contract system, 124
Couvade, 26-27
Covert sensitization, 125
Crossover studies, 54-55, 83-84, 107,
    133
Cultural factors, 26-27
Cumulative effect, xv

D-amphetamine sulphate (AMP), 18
Darvon, 29, 31
Definitions, xii-xv
Demand characteristics, 40, 93-96,
    115-116, 121-122
Depression, 47-49, 107-108, 130
Desensitization, 121-122
Diagnostic and Statistical Manual
    (American Psychiatric Association),
    44
Diazepam, 29, 82-85
Double-blind procedure, xiv, 19, 29,
    46, 103, 126, 132-135
Drug efficiency index, 31-32
Drug research, 126, 132-133

Ecological validity, 24, 39-40, 61, 79,
    82, 88, 96
Electric shocks, 101-102
Emotion, theory of, 143-144

"Environmental set," 96
Ephedrine, 51
Epinephrine, 86
Ether, 26
Ethyl crotyl barbituate, 18
Expectations, 80, 104-106; about goal attainment, 139-142; of symptom reduction, 116-117
Experimental analogue, 39-40

Familiarity variable, 99
Field dependency, 66, 75
Fluphenazine, 45, 46
Folk medicine, 1-5
Frustration tests, 121-122

General adaptation syndrome (GAS), 37
"General Attitude Variability Inventory" (GAVI), 64
Ginseng, 4
Gliceryl trinitrate, 19
Goal achievement motivation, 139-142
Great Britain, 107
GSR, 66

Hallucination, 9-10
Hallucinogenic drugs, 22-25, 65
Hathaway coding system, 62
Hawthorne effect, 130
Health, illness, and sick-role behavior, 35-36, 38-39
"Hello-goodbye" pattern, 115-116
Hippocrates, 5
"Hope," 139-143
Huang-ti, 4
Hypnosis, 29, 76-77, 87-88

"Iatroplacebogenics," 104
Imipramine, 107
Independent assessment team (IAT), 134-135
Indian medicine, 4
"Individual"/"group" experiments, 68-69
Insight-oriented therapy, 122-123
Instructional sets, 96, 99-101

Interior/exterior body regions, 85, 86
Introversion, 67, 69-70
Ischemic muscle pain, 29-30

James-Lange theory of emotion, 143-144
Japanese medicine, 5

Learning theory, 10-11
Librium, 55, 81-82
Lysergic acid diethylamide (LSD-25), 22-24, 51, 66, 74

Marijuana, 24-25
Medicine and surgery, 41-43
Meprobamate, 21, 55, 70, 74, 105-106, 108
Methodological problems, 129-135
Methylamphetamine, 114
Metronidazole, 52
MMPI, 63-64, 68, 81
Morphine, 26, 31, 71, 72

Negative placebo effect. See Nocebo effect
Negative placebo reactors and nonreactors, 60-61
Negative placebos. See Nocebos
Nei-Ching ("The Theory of Internal Diseases"), 4
Neurotics: as placebo reactors, 67, 69, 99-100; vs. psychotics as negative reactors, 60, 102; and therapist personality, 105-106
No-treatment controls, 129-130
Nocebo effect, xiv, 82
Nocebos, xiv, 22, 52
Nonpatients: and nonprojective personality instruments, 62-70; vs. patients in tests, 40, 61, 82, 86, 88, 96; as placebo reactors, 89
Nonprojective personality instruments, 62-70
Nurses, 103

"Open trial," 42

Pain, 25-33, 64-65, 71-72
Patient/nonpatient experiments, 40, 61, 86, 90, 96
Patients as subjects, 70-75
Pentobarbital, 98
Perphenazine, 53
Personality and Healing (Frank), 35
Personality questionnaire, 80-82
Personality vs. environmental variables, 91
Phenobarbital, 55, 105-106, 108
Phenobarbitone, 107
Phenothiazines, 45-46
"Phenotypic"/"genotypic" characteristics, 77
Physical contact theory (PCT), 124-125
Physiological/psychological arousal, 100-102, 144-145
Placebo, defined, xii-xiii, 119, 126
Placebo analgesia, 28-33, 42
Placebo color and taste, 11-13
Placebo controls, 122-127
Placebo dependence, xv, 44
Placebo effect: defined, xiii-xiv, 93, 112; review of the literature, xv-xvii
Placebo-proneness of psychological functions, 21-22
Placebo reactivity/resistance, 24, 29, 53-54
Placebo reactors, personality of, 59-92, 119-120; nonprojective personality instruments, 62-70; projective personality instruments, 70-75; suggestibility/acquiescence hypothesis, 75-88
Placebo response, defined, xiii
Placebogenic variables, defined, xiv
Placebos, parenteral vs. oral, 13-14
Placebos et effet placebo en médecine (Kissel and Barrucand), xvi, 42
Positive placebo effect. *See* Placebo effect
"Positive placebo response," 56
Pretests, 130-132
Prochlorperazine, 44
Prognostic uses of placebos, 53-57

Prognostigenic variables, xiv
Projective personality instruments, 70-75
Psychiatry, 43-57
Psychoanalytic theory, 9-10
"Psychological distress," 36-39
Psychology of hope, 139-142
Psychology of illness: review of the literature, 36-37
Psychophysiological and psychometric tests, 20-22, 96
Psychotherapy, 109-127
Psychotics vs. neurotics as negative reactors, 60, 102
Psychotomimetic drugs, 68
Psychotropic drugs, 68
Public speaking anxiety, 122-123
Puzzle of Pain (Melzack), 26

Race differences, 42, 45
Randomization design, 130, 131
Rational-emotive therapy (RET), 123-124
Rauwolfia, 4
Referral source for therapy, 116-117
Rehospitalization, 46
Relaxation treatment, 121-122, 123
Religion and medicine, 2
Religiousness, 73, 90
Remission, spontaneous, 47, 48, 49
Response sets, 80-82
Role expectations, 93, 96
Rorschach test, 71, 72, 74

Schizophrenics, 13, 14, 43-47, 53, 102, 124
Scopolamine, 17
Self-awareness, 145-146
Self-control, 124, 125
Sensation threshold, 27
Sex differences, 45, 86
Single-blind procedure, xiv, 126
Situational analysis, 91, 93-108, 144-145
Smoking behavior, 125
Soldiers, wounded, 27
Soviet Union, 51

State/trait variables, 29, 30, 74, 87
Stimulants, 18, 96-97, 98
Stimuli, outer/inner, 75
Stress, psychological/system, 36-39
Suggestibility, 19, 42, 75-79, 87-88, 143
Susruta Samhita, 4
Symptom distress groups, 120-121
Symptom reduction, 116-117, 118
Systematic desensitization, 121-124, 125

TAT, 71, 72
Tetrahydrocannabinols (THC), 25
"Theory of Internal Diseases" (*Nei-Ching*), 4
Therapist, personality of, 102-108
Therapy, physical/psychic, xi, 5-8, 15, 102, 106, 147-148
Thermal sensitivity, 28
Thiopentone, 114
Thioridazine, 44, 45, 46

Thorazine, 67, 96
Time-effect curve, xv
Tolerance sensitivity, xv
Trance induction procedure, 88
Tranquilizers, 18, 44, 50, 68, 87, 96-97, 98, 133
Triple-blind procedure, xiv, 60

Ultrasonic stimulation, 28, 64

Varieties of Religious Experience (James), 76
Verbal-oriented therapy (VOT), 124-125
Volunteer/nonvolunteer subjects, 63
Voodoo, 38, 90

WAIS, 71, 72, 74
Weight loss, 124
Wounds, soldier/civilian, 27

Xylocaine, 97

About the Author

Michael Jospe was born in South Africa and received his undergraduate education at the University of the Witwatersrand, Johannesburg, and the University of Leeds, England. He received the Ph.D. in psychology from the University of Minnesota in Minneapolis. He is particularly interested in multi-disciplinary approaches to a number of medical and psychiatric problems, and in the role that clinical psychologists can play as part of the health care team. Formerly chief psychologist at Newington Children's Hospital in Newington, Connecticut, he is now in private practice in Los Angeles, California.